The Iron Edge

For improved memory, learning, energy, mood, impulse control, and general health

by

Ron Hoggan, Ed. D.

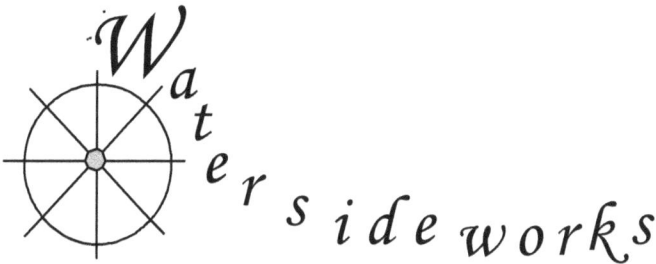

Watersideworks

VIDEO, E-CARD AND PRINT PUBLICATIONS

www.waterside-works.com

1988 Falcon Crescent RR - 1

Cowichan Bay, B.C., Canada

V0R 1N1

I am indebted to the many people who have helped me structure the contents of this book with their helpful criticism, artfulness, and thoughtful commentary. These include, but are not limited to, my wife, Betty, Tony Allen, Bob Machon, teachers who attended my lectures to the Calgary City Teachers' Convention, 2008. I am also grateful for the considerable encouragement and support from colleagues, Sandi Nichol, Jim Stevenson, Pat Cyca, Colin Hill, and countless students. I thank you all.

Author's note:

My field is Education. I have spent the last 20 years teaching high school students. I spent about half of that time working with special and/or reluctant students.

On a personal level, I have also struggled with iron deficiency for as long as I can remember. During that time I heard many explanations from a variety of health care professionals. They made sense to me at the time. Each was subsequently proven incorrect or at least, very unlikely. Other, perhaps wiser, physicians dodged my questions. Despite many apparently good ideas, every suggestion, postulation, and explanation proved ineffective, incorrect, or both.

I quit smoking cigarettes, as my GP felt that might be a factor in many of my health problems, including my iron deficiency. I increased my meat consumption. I took vitamin C supplements. None of these seemed to help my iron status. Then, in 1994, I was diagnosed with celiac disease. I thought that I finally had an answer. But my iron deficiency persisted despite a very strict gluten-free diet over all the years since my diagnosis. I ate more meat. Still, my test results continued to reveal iron deficiency. For some time now, I have controlled my iron with iron supplements. However, I am now applying the principles explained in this book, and it appears that I no longer need iron supplements.

It was not until I began my own search of the medical literature, in pursuit of my doctoral degree in Education, that I found some answers that have proven helpful to my iron status challenges. For instance, I learned that many features of my lifestyle worsened my iron status. Despite my iron-rich diet, excessive consumption of coffee, along with many of my food preferences and eating habits, interfered with my ability to absorb iron. To make matters worse, I have a sweet tooth. My inclination is to displace healthier foods with ones that fulfill my cravings for sweets and pastries.

I began my research into iron metabolism to learn about its impact on learning and behavior but I soon learned what I needed to do to correct my iron problems. The central focus of this book is on the cognitive side of iron's many functions in the human body and brain. However, given my personal interest in the subject, and since it is almost impossible to deal with iron's impact on memory and learning in isolation, *Get the Iron Edge* also explores many other contributions that iron makes to human wellness. Iron's impact on immune function, growth, and strength are important, relevant issues and are also discussed throughout this book. Nonetheless, it is my personal experiences along with the interaction between iron metabolism and various educational concerns including memory, deductive/analytical skills, ability to pay attention, learn, and remember that have shaped and informed my understanding of this subject.

Get the Iron Edge is composed of information I have assembled that will be helpful to anyone who is interested in managing their iron status regardless of their motives. My goal is to assist readers in knowledgeably achieving and maintaining a healthy iron status just as I have done. The pursuit of this goal will ultimately lead to optimizing your learning capacity, memory, educational opportunities, vocational endeavors, parenting skills, intellectual growth, and general health, while learning about new scientific developments in this exciting area of wellness research..

It should be noted, however, that this book is not relevant to forms of anemia that are not caused by iron deficiency. Neither is it relevant to such hereditary iron deficiency conditions as thalassemia.

In keeping with the perspective that each of us must take control of our own health care, *Get the Iron Edge* is aimed at developing a context in which readers will have the opportunity to explore the controversies related to learning, education, and iron deficiency. Based on data from human and animal studies that have been published in the peer reviewed medical literature, I have drawn information about these issues, and attempted to evaluate their relative merits and weaknesses. Still, it is up to individual readers and their health care professionals to determine specific, individual iron needs, and act accordingly. Appropriate testing and clinical assessment are critical to effective, appropriate health care in relation to iron status.

Formatting note:

In order to save space I have just listed the first author's last name within brackets then I have alphabetized the list of sources for ease of reference. This is not, to my knowledge, a standard approach, but I thought it would be easiest for readers.

Table of Contents

Chapter One Introduction   8
A Promise
Iron deficiency is entirely too common
Iron deficiency with and without anemia
Iron toxicity
Testing
What this book offers to readers
A caveat

Chapter Two How we gain and lose iron   15
How we absorb iron
How we lose iron
Iron absorption rates
Cultural practices and social status
Factors that inhibit iron absorption
Inhibitors of non-heme iron absorption (table 1)
Socio-economic status
The dairy myth
Nutritional miscues threaten our children
Nutritoxicity in need of a name
Illness
Rheumatoid arthritis
Malignant disease

Chapter Three Who is at risk and why?   22
Signs and symptoms of iron deficiency
What problems are caused by iron deficiency?
General classes of risk groups
Specific risk groups I
nfants and children
Adolescents
Pregnant or lactating women
Athletes
What about body builders?
First Nations communities
Vegetarians
Other lifestyle choices & dietary practices

From fetus to old age
Factors that inhibit iron absorption
Iron as a function of social status
Cultural risk factors
Additional nutritional risk factors

Chapter Four Optimizing Absorption

Heme and non-heme iron
Comparative absorption rates for heme and non-heme iron (table 2)
Factors that aid iron absorption
Stomach acid
Combined consumption of heme and non-heme iron
Dietary factors that enhance absorption of iron (table 3)
A few sources of non-heme iron
Heme iron
Supplements

Chapter Five Some basics of iron metabolism

Synthesis of hemoglobin and its function
ATP synthesis, muscle metabolism, and energy conversion
Iron's importance to neurotransmitter synthesis and function
Iron's involvement in myelin formation Iron deficiency can alter insulin sensitivity and mood

Chapter Six Iron status and learning

Iron deficiency and the brain
Three theories about how iron causes cognitive problems
Iron deficient infants
Menstruation, Mathematics, and iron
My classroom experience
How students respond to iron supplements
Some of the controversies
Some incomplete answers
Harnessing the controversies

Chapter Seven What tests to request and how to interpret the results
Measurements of the various forms of iron in the body (table 4)
Normal values for hemoglobin (table 5)

Chapter Eight Relevant nutritional controversies
Whose dietary advice can we trust?
How do these recommendations impact on iron status?
Should the food pyramid be changed?

Chapter Nine Iron overload
What is overload?
Symptoms of overload
Diagnosing iron overload
Advanced cases of overload

Chapter Ten Conclusion
Further research is needed
The peer review process
Patient self-management
Education

CHAPTER ONE

Introduction

A Promise

The title of this book implies a promise. It suggests that by following the instructions and suggestions provided here, you will develop an intellectual and physical advantage. That promise is true for anyone who is at risk of developing, or is currently experiencing, iron deficiency. Since almost every one of us, at some stage of our lives, has been, or will be, at risk of developing iron deficiency, this book offers an advantage or potential advantage to almost every individual who reads it. In addition to improving your own physical and intellectual function, if and when iron deficiency threatens, it will also help you to become a better parent, teacher, and consumer of foods and food services.

Iron is a widely accepted, traditional metaphor for strength. This analogy extends right into the present day and deeply into the human body and brain. In order to grow and become stronger, our muscles need a great deal of iron. For that matter, any tissue growth requires iron. Human strength also lies in our ability to fight disease, to think and act quickly, avoid hazards, process sensory input, assess risks, communicate, cooperate, and recall hazardous situations. Iron is a necessary component of all of these dimensions of human strength. Whether we are talking about our ancient cave-dwelling ancestors or today's apartment-dwelling urbanites, the power of iron helps us to survive, thrive, and procreate.

Iron deficiency is entirely too common

Yet iron deficiency, with and without anemia, is a worldwide problem that afflicts large portions of every population of the world, at various stages of many individuals' lives. As one group of medical researchers put it, "Disturbances of iron metabolism, particularly iron deficiency and iron redistribution are among the most commonly overlooked or misinterpreted diseases" (Wick). This may be due, in large part at least, to a common failure to recognize the importance and hazards of iron deficiency and iron overload.

It may surprise you to learn that iron deficiency is even common in industrialized nations, where our affluence offers us a very wide range of rich sources of nutritional iron. Nonetheless, iron deficiency afflicts approximately one quarter of menstruating women in the United States (de Benoist) (Ames). A condition of low iron stores, which usually develops prior to anemia, and is thus likely to be more common, is frequently found among adolescent girls and young women in the US who are still attending school.

Of course, residents of developing nations experience an even greater risk of this very common nutrient deficiency (Hashizume). Inadequate food supply is just one of many factors causing this deficiency. For instance, intestinal parasite infections common to the third world also cause excessive iron losses, further exacerbating the iron status problems among these disadvantaged people. Iron deficiency is a worldwide challenge.

Iron deficiency with and without anemia

Some contend that iron deficiency anemia is the most important manifestation of iron deficiency. However, as you will learn in Chapter 5, most of the symptoms of compromised cognitive function appear in the context of low iron stores, and long before the onset of anemia.

Sometimes iron deficiency can cause anemia, which compromises our ability to distribute oxygen to all the cells in our bodies and brains. In other cases, iron deficiency may only show up as a shortage of iron stores, usually indicated by ferritin levels. Iron deficiency anemia is often assumed to be accompanied by low ferritin levels. However, some people exhibit anemia despite sufficient or even elevated levels of ferritin. Deficiencies in either hemoglobin or iron stores can be a serious problem that is often accompanied by very troubling signs and symptoms. Ignoring either form of iron deficiency is a serious mistake.

Iron toxicity

Too much iron can also cause serious health problems, especially when iron in the bloodstream exceeds the amount of available transferrin and ferritin. This is partly because bacteria need iron to reproduce. In addition to the many other hazards it poses, free iron can provide a fertile context for bacterial infections to multiply rapidly and quickly get out of control. Another important consideration is a condition of iron overload which can cause very disturbing symptoms, give rise to serious ailments, injure the liver, heart, and other vital organs and in rare cases, cause premature death. A more detailed discussion of this issue is provided in chapter nine, but it still falls far short of a comprehensive explanation. Thus, if you have concerns in this area, you would be well advised to seek additional, more complete sources of information.

Testing

One of the most important elements of the message offered here is that appropriate laboratory testing is a critically important tool for managing iron metabolism. Very serious, dangerous mistakes can arise out of beginning to supplement iron out of a desire to take a short-cut to improved intellectual functioning. Chapter seven outlines the importance of testing, how to interpret test results, and what actions may be taken. It is important to have a clear destination in mind before beginning a journey. It is also important to have a clear objective when attempting to manage your iron metabolism. Appropriate testing is the best aid for determining your goal and avoiding some significant hazards that can arise from excessive iron.

What this book offers to readers

Get the Iron Edge is a guide to help the reader to regain or achieve optimal physical, immunological, and intellectual function through optimizing iron stores and hemoglobin without compromising absorption of other minerals. It shows readers how and why iron deficiencies develop, the potential consequences of these conditions and, most importantly, how to identify and correct these problems through altering lifestyle choices and other conditions that are interfering with optimal iron status. It also provides a brief, limited explanation of iron overload as it is a very important concern. Unfortunately, the author is not well versed in this area.

A caveat

As with any claim based on scientific research, what we know today is always under revision as new discoveries arise to change our thinking. Thus, the advice offered in this book is open to revision as new information becomes available. This is a plain language reflection of my understanding of current knowledge in the realm of iron metabolism and cognitive function.

In the next chapter we will start to examine iron metabolism issues in detail. We will explore how we gain and lose iron and why these issues are of importance.

CHAPTER TWO

How we gain and lose iron

How we absorb iron

Through chewing, the actions of saliva, and digestive acids, the mouth and stomach break down proteins that are bound to iron. An enzyme called ferric reductase alters ferric iron to ferrous iron which is the only form in which it can be absorbed. The ferrous iron is then moved into a cell. A special protein (DMT1) transports most minerals across the membrane of cells that line the intestinal wall. If the iron is then bound to ferritin, that iron will remain in the cell and be wasted in fecal matter when the cell dies. (These cells are replaced every few days so this is an important facet of iron loss.) More often, the iron will bind to a ferroportin protein and move from the cell into the bloodstream.

How we lose iron

We lose iron in our sweat, in fecal matter (as mentioned above) through menstruation, through inflammation, and through any form of injury or illness that causes blood loss. As you will soon learn, this list is deceptively short. There are many, many ways in which we can lose iron. Some detail is provided on the major causes of iron loss but the subject is enormous and detailed exploration is beyond the scope of this book.

Iron absorption rates

Most of us can meet our iron needs if we absorb about 1 mg. each day. However, adolescents, pregnant or lactating women, and menstruating women all require about

5 mg per day. Athletes will vary in their requirements, depending on the extent of their exertions. Children and infants' needs are equally variable according to their current growth rates.

Cultural practices and social status

Unfortunately, coffee and tea consumption have become so ingrained in our culture that most of us drink one of these beverages during or immediately after each meal. In doing so, we unwittingly inhibit our absorption of iron and other minerals from the food we have just eaten. Such practices are particularly problematic for those with additional risk factors for mineral deficiencies.

The polyphenols in coffee and teas have been identified as the culprits that interfere with iron absorption. They bind to iron making it unavailable for absorption, thus reducing it to a useless waste product. When taken with or immediately after a meal, these drinks can have a very damaging impact on our iron status, yet when taken more than an hour prior or two hours after eating, they can be relatively harmless in this regard.

Factors that inhibit iron absorption

As mentioned above, cow and goat milk consumption can inhibit iron absorption. Another common cause of iron malabsorption is reduced stomach acids. The many commercials for over-the-counter anti-acids suggest that sales are booming in this area. It is my experience that food allergies, gluten sensitivity, and celiac disease are often at the root of excessive gastric acidity. However, these anti-acid products along with acid blocking prescription medications will interfere with iron absorption. Low vitamin C status will also inhibit iron absorption.

Coffee, black tea, whole grains, legumes, and nuts will all interfere with iron absorption through binding to iron in a way that is not reversible by digestion.

It should be borne in mind that calcium intake will inhibit both heme and non-heme iron absorption (Lynch). It does this by competing for transport through the cell wall.

Table 1

Inhibitors of non-heme iron absorption.

Polyphenols	black tea, herb teas, coffee, cocoa, some grain products, red wine
Phytate	Whole grains, legumes (peas, beans and lentils), soybeans, rice
Oxalate	spinach, chard, beet greens, rhubarb, sweet potato
Non-phytate component of soy protein	soy protein
Calcium	food and supplements

(from Pasut, L., 2002)

Socio-economic status

Inadequate consumption of iron-rich foods is yet another important factor in iron deficiency (Bruner). Poverty often dictates a diet that contains little bioavailable iron along with many antinutrients such as phytates found in grains and legumes, as well as the inhibition of iron absorption caused by dairy products – another group of poverty foods.

The dairy myth

Walter Willet, among others, has written extensively to dispel the myth that dairy consumption is a healthful practice. He has highlighted the fallacy of cow's milk consumption and the highly bioavailable calcium that is so often touted as beneficial, and shown that regular dairy consumption does not prevent fractures. There is good evidence that cow's milk does interfere with iron absorption. Cow's milk will induce anemia in infants by causing increased intestinal blood losses. There is also reason to suspect that lactoferrin, a protein found in cow's milk, will play a role in inducing anemia. Later in life, calcium rich dairy products will cause an imbalance when competing with other minerals for absorption across the intestinal barrier. The sought-after benefits of improved calcium absorption will be offset by inhibition of absorption of other equally important minerals.

The oxalates found in a variety of vegetables, as listed in table 1, can also inhibit iron absorption and should be consumed in moderation.

Nutritional miscues threaten our children

Iron deficiency is widespread among the children and adolescents in industrialized nations, where iron-rich food is available in abundance. Therefore, iron education programs may provide rapid social change and extensive human and economic benefits. An important factor in widespread iron deficiency is the cacophony of competing nutritional ideologies that surround conventional nutritional wisdom. For instance, healthy eating guides such as the USDA food guide, and other such literature tend to lag far behind relevant scientific findings, often as a result of pressures from competing economic and political interests.

For instance, many of us believe we should feed cow's milk and rice pabulum to infants who are beginning to eat solid food. However, this feeding practice is particularly likely to cause iron deficiency. Although rice has a low rate of inciting allergies, it contains two potent anti-nutrients, in the form of polyphenols and phytates that interfere with iron absorption. Add to this, the independent risk for iron depletion posed by milk, and it is not difficult to see the problem posed by this feeding practice, and iron is not the only mineral at issue here.

Unfortunately, feeding milk and rice pabulum continues to be recommended to new parents by health care professionals based on traditional notions that run contrary to the relevant research. Such feeding often begins at about six months of age, when iron stores from the womb are typically depleted, and considerable iron is needed to sustain the continuing rapid growth typical of this stage of life. Such feeding practices are of special concern in infants who were less than full-term because it is in the very late stages of pregnancy when unborn babies are accruing the bulk of their iron stores to sustain them until they can get iron from solid foods. Breast milk typically supplies negligible amounts of iron.

Research findings that should inform our perspectives on these issues are often lost amid the voices of well financed lobbyists and special interest groups that can dominate the media and the political scene, these powerful forces have been reported as being exerted on the USDA's food guide (Nestle).

Nutritoxicity in need of a name

In a more general sense, there is something of an invisible linguistic barrier that is raised against the systematic study and understanding of nutrition-driven disease. Some forms of illness that are caused by nutritional miscues have been successfully treated for centuries. For instance, long before we understood vitamin C, or its importance to our good health, British sailors became known as "Limeys" for their consumption of limes to stave off scurvy. (More recent research shows that limes are a comparatively poor source of vitamin C.)

Yet we have no name for these diseases that arise from nutritional deficiencies and the mistaken nutritional beliefs that often drive them. We have a name for diseases caused by flawed or misguided medical treatment. These diseases are lumped together under the term "iatrogenic illness" (Cook,). When our immune systems turn against us, we call these ailments "autoimmune diseases." Such terms confer a legitimizing aura on their subject. Thus, I propose that a descriptive term be coined to identify and classify the wide range of ailments including cases of iron deficiency and iron deficie0ncy anemia that result from institutionalized nutritional errors. One term that might be considered is "nutritoxic." It captures the notion that a nutritional error contributes to or causes the illnesses. .

Illness

A variety of illnesses can also induce iron deficiency. It is often an important indictor of disease, injury, or atypical blood loss and may be the first of a series of signs that will lead physicians to any of a number of diagnoses. For instance, celiac disease is a very common cause of unexplained iron deficiency. A vast majority of individuals with celiac disease do not know they have an illness and will often fail to learn about it until one of the cancers associated with celiac disease is diagnosed. Some evidence suggests that iron is not well absorbed through the intestinal wall in people with celiac disease. Other evidence suggests that intestinal inflammation and fecal blood losses are causative factors. It may be that all three abnormalities contribute to iron deficiencies found very commonly in people with untreated celiac disease. Similar dynamics are at work in many intestinal diseases including Crohn's, colitis, and diverticulitis, where iron deficiency abounds. Yet those who suffer from these ailments are frequently told to follow government sanctioned eating guides that promote excessive grain and dairy consumption. This advice runs contrary to a burgeoning body of research evidence amassed over the last two or three decades.

Rheumatoid arthritis

Rheumatoid arthritis is another ailment that causes iron deficiency. Here, it is the inflammatory process that is usually blamed for most of the iron losses. Many ailments, especially autoimmune diseases, are also characterized by iron metabolism errors, including hemochromatosis, which is a condition of iron overload (more on this later).

Malignant disease

Tumours require large supplies of iron and they will pre-empt other body systems to meet their iron needs. This is yet another reason why regular iron testing can be valuable. It can provide an early warning of hazards that might otherwise escape detection for some time. Free iron is especially problematic when tumours are present, as the free iron is highly available to promote tissue growth in the tumour.

Now we will look at who is at greater risk of developing iron deficiency, and what signs and symptoms to look for in these individuals.

CHAPTER THREE

Who is at risk and why?

Signs and symptoms of iron deficiency

Poor intellectual performance is both a common finding, and an important cause for concern in iron deficiency but there are many other signs and symptoms that should alert us to the possibility of a shortage of this mineral. These signs and symptoms include crankiness, poor impulse control, fatigue, depression, indifference, restlessness, inattention, hyperactivity (which is especially common in iron deficient children and adolescents) or under-activity, poor concentration, inattention, reversal of normal sleep-wake patterns (shift to a nocturnal schedule and daytime sleeping) compulsively eating ice, and pica (eating non-food substances such as dirt, wood, paint, etc.). Any one or more of the foregoing, in the absence of a good explanation, should raise concern about iron deficiency and testing should be undertaken as soon as possible.

What problems are caused by iron deficiency?

Some of the problems that come from iron deficiency will be obvious from the signs and symptoms listed above. Other hazards may be less obvious. For instance, pica is a particularly hazardous eating disorder in infants and children who live or play in older buildings where paint may contain lead. Chewing on painted surfaces may release paint that is swallowed along with the lead it contains. Thus, in addition to their current state of iron deficiency, children with pica are also at risk of developing lead poisoning, which is all too common among inner-city children. In addition to the mental retardation that often accompanies iron deficiencies at critical stages of infancy and early childhood, lead toxicity is also a risk factor for irreversible mental retardation.

Iron deficiency can have other serious health implications as well. Inattention, indifference, and fatigue are not helpful to children who have to cross busy thoroughfares. The same traits in adult drivers can have similarly disastrous consequences. Crankiness, hyperactivity, and restlessness can also lead to rash behaviors and serious accidents. Iron deficiency frequently leads to reduced impulse control which can pose a variety of problems – road rage comes immediately to mind.

Iron deficiency will also increase susceptibility to inflammation due to the importance of iron to our immune systems. For instance, iron deficiency causes a decrease in the anti-inflammatory action of interleukin 2 (IL2) while simultaneously causing an increase in pro-inflammatory Interleukin 1 (IL1).

Iron deficiency also increases the likelihood of hearing loss by making auditory nerves more susceptible to damage.

In addition to the above, a host of health problems can arise out of ccompromised oxygen distribution. Iron is necessary for hemoglobin production in the bone marrow, and is critical to the assimilation, distribution, and release of oxygen at the appropriate times and places within the body.

General classes of risk groups

Iron deficiency can strike almost anyone but here is a set of general categories that signal a greater risk:

1. gender
2. rapid tissue growth;
3. injury;
4. inadequate iron absorption, and;
5. Illness.
6.

Specific risk groups:

Infants and children experiencing phases of rapid growth, adolescents, pregnant or lactating women, vegetarians, members of First Nations communities, and endurance athletes all experience an increased risk of developing iron deficiency (Zlotkin). Several common ailments and diseases also increase the risk of developing iron deficiency (Swanson,). Excessive loss through bleeding and/or through impaired absorption of iron can also deplete iron stores (Bruner) and different risk factors for iron deficiency arise at various stages of life.

Infants and children

Infants and children frequently experience periods of rapid growth. Infants have a very limited ability to absorb iron. It is often difficult, without a concerted effort, to keep pace with these periodic increases in their iron needs. Many pediatricians prescribe iron supplements immediately after birth, continuing until solid foods are started. Growing larger tissues involves increased cellular reproduction which places large demands on iron stores. Added to depleting iron stores are the proportional iron losses due to the increasing volume of blood. As children grow, they have increasing blood volumes and iron absorption must keep pace with this dual demand for more iron to support tissue growth along with greater iron requirements due to increased blood volume. Thus, infants and children have a particularly large and important need for iron, and concerned parents should try to ensure adequate iron intake and absorption especially during growth spurts.

Adolescents

Adolescent males are frequently caught in a multiple bind when it comes to meeting their iron needs. They are growing muscle and bone tissues very quickly. Puberty is taking its toll through iron use in all the processes associated with this dramatic change in body conformation, including increased hormone and enzyme production. Adolescence is also a time when many become quite involved in sports. Further, common dietary practices at this stage of life are potentially disastrous. Sugar and junk food appear to be the mainstay of many adolescent diets. All of these forces combine to make adolescence a time when iron repletion seems more of a fortuitous accident.

Adolescent females are in an even worse position when it comes to their iron status. In addition to all of the above issues faced by males, although female growth usually slows sometime after the onset of menses, all of the other factors are dwarfed by the large iron losses that occur with menstruation.

Thus, adolescence is a time of excessive and variable risk for iron deficiency. This is an age group where poor school performance and poor impulse control may be compounding other behavioral challenges common to this age group. Some researchers report iron deficiency at 39% among teenage girls (Gibson).

Such high levels of iron deficiency are concentrated among high risk groups such as disadvantaged children, adolescents, and adults. Nonetheless, such dramatic findings suggest a need for individuals to take control of this important health and learning issue. Large U.S. studies show that 23% of males and 18% of females aged 2 to 18 years, do not consume recommended levels of meat and other foods required to maintain a healthy iron status (Putnam) while other reports indicate a rate of iron deficiency anemia in excess of 14% among adolescent girls in the U.S. (Institute of Medicine). Similarly, a 14% rate of iron deficiency has been reported among teen-aged girls in Sweden (Samuelson).

Pregnant or lactating women

Similarly, pregnant or lactating women are extremely iron challenged. When their iron is not lost to menstruation, women of child bearing age are passing iron along to the fetus they are carrying. Under ideal circumstances, the fetus will store enough iron during the final six weeks of pregnancy to meet the vast majority of its iron needs until about 6 months of age when she/he will begin to get iron from solid foods. Thus, premature infants are particularly likely to be iron deficient as they have missed some or all of these final weeks in the womb when the fetus absorbs much of the mother's stored iron. More than 20% of the pregnant women studied in the U.S. had iron deficiency anemia, while more than 40% had some degree of iron deficiency (Swensen).

One report (Pasut) indicates that iron status early in pregnancy has the strongest influence on birth outcomes. Hence, Pasut argues for improvement of iron status prior to pregnancy. She goes on to identify schools as a potential avenue for reaching adolescent girls in order to reduce rates of anemia and iron deficiency prior to pregnancy.

Although very little iron is passed to the infant in the mother's milk, she is still using considerable amounts of iron during lactation and is at particular risk of developing iron deficiency since her iron stores will have been seriously depleted late in the pregnancy.

Athletes

Athletes, particularly those involved in endurance sports, are another group that experience a significant risk of iron deficiency. Again, because of menstruation, females may have greater cause for concern when engaged in endurance athletics although there is some evidence to suggest a converging risk (see section on body builders). Any time we are growing new tissues, iron is used. We also lose iron through perspiration, urine, and feces. Athletes can be expected to continuously build muscle, repair injured tissues, and perspire a great deal. Yet about 30% of the female athletes at Auburn University were found to consume diets that contained inadequate quantities of iron (Gropper). Athletes should be particularly concerned about maintaining optimal iron levels to ensure their best performance and to avoid the many other hazards of iron deficiency.

What about body builders?

Although the research regarding iron status in connection with weight training/body building is sparse, it appears that women may enjoy some advantages for conserving their iron stores while involved in these activities. The research group led by Deruisseau showed that while hemoglobin levels dropped in both gender groups of weight training athletes, only the men experienced drops in ferritin levels. While the above research does not appear to have been replicated, published research in this area is sparse and such reports should be given due consideration while we await further investigations of this issue.

First Nations communities

First Nations communities appear to experience a very high risk of iron deficiency. This may well be due to their recent adoption of European dietary practices. They are newcomers to consuming cereal grains, legumes, dairy products, and refined carbohydrates (sugar, syrup, etc.). All of these relatively new foods, which we are now learning can be very harmful to the people who consume them, may be especially harmful to those whose genetic background has not prepared them for such eating practices. (Although a mere hiccup in evolutionary terms, those of European descent have had at least a few centuries and possibly as much as several millennia to adapt to such a diet.) Levels of iron deficiency are reported as 38% among Inuit infants at 12 months of age (Willows).

Vegetarians

I am awed by nature's beauty when I see a majestic buck sporting a large rack and strutting confidently through the woods. I am also moved by the harsh and inhumane practices that are part of every feed lot I have seen. How, then can I attack the eating practices of those who are so touched by these same issues and similar concerns about these beautiful animals and our sometimes bestial carnivorous practices? I may not agree with the vegetarian perspective on a nutritional level, but I find it exceedingly difficult to disagree with their ethics.

In addition to encouraging vegetarians to ensure they have adequate vitamin B12 intakes, either through supplements or consumption of some animal products (some do consume eggs or fish) I want to encourage vegetarians to read on and learn about how they can maximize their iron absorption through harnessing non-heme sources of iron.

Other lifestyle choices & dietary practices

Even apparently irrelevant dietary practices can impact on our iron status. The last decade or so has seen an exponential increase in awareness of the health hazards of cereal grain consumption. Here is yet another facet of this widespread nutritional miscue. Consumption of grain products can induce iron deficiency through binding of parts of the grain, called phytates, and subsequent wasting of that complex. The bound iron might otherwise have been absorbed (de Benoist) (Cordain).

The following statement is both representative of the views of researchers in this area, and possibly quite surprising to those who eat what they consider to be a healthy diet: "Typical grain- based or rice-based complimentary foods are poor sources of iron and may contain phytic acid which is a potent inhibitor of iron absorption." (Zlotkin). Many other authorities in this area have voiced similar concerns about our increasing reliance upon grains as the foundation of our modern diet (Cordain, 1999) ((Hashizume) (Pilu) (Duhan) (Layrisse) (Tseng).

Although whole grains do have a lower rating on the glycemic index, they are also loaded with phytates. A variety of beans, seeds, and nuts also contain considerable quantities of phytates. We humans, as opposed to ruminants, do not have the necessary digestive enzymes to break the bond that forms between minerals and phytates. Thus, when we eat these foods, our digestive tracts provide an ideal environment for these bonds to form, ultimately leading to the wasting of important minerals that might have benefitted us enormously.

This quality of phytates is why they are sometimes called anti-nutrients. Polyphenols and oxalates can also act as anti-nutrients that interfere with non-heme iron absorption.

Similarly, there is also some unknown factor in soy protein that inhibits non-heme iron absorption, although calcium is currently the only known inhibitor that interferes with the absorption of both types of iron. (See table 1.)

From fetus to old age

Individual iron requirements vary across different stages of life, and according to gender, activity levels, dietary habits, iron losses, wellness and a host of other factors. Regular testing of ferritin, hemoglobin, and transferrin is our best way of telling whether our needs are being met, identifying problems and how to correct those problems. Recent research shows that 9% of apparently healthy seniors are iron deficient (Roebothan) and that study excluded seniors with any of the ailments that would predispose to iron deficiencies such as rheumatoid arthritis. Iron is also one of the several minerals that have been implicated in some investigations of Alzheimer's disease (Finefrock).

Iron as a function of social status

One group (Yu.) has argued that education is unlikely to have any important impact in the realm of iron deficiency because it is a condition that is largely conferred by one's socio-economic status. Yet, one of the cornerstones of public education, in the context of a democracy, is to provide opportunities for all citizens to participate fully in their culture and government. Implicit in this proposition is the possibility, perhaps even the expectation, of upward social mobility. Thus, an iron sufficiency instructional program may be an important tool for educators to use in aiding students' upward social mobility. If students can take control of their iron status, they may aid both their learning today and their prosperity tomorrow.

Iron instruction also offers benefits to those who occupy a more advantaged economic position. Despite claims that iron deficiency is a function of socio-economic status, or is simply the result of poor dietary choices (Butriss) this nutrient deficiency is widespread even among the affluent populations of the industrialized world (Kretchmer) (Bruner) (Caballero).

In further contradiction of some such claims that either blame the victims for poor dietary choices, or for their social status, it may be that poor dietary choices are better described as ill-informed choices. Healthy eating guides continue to advocate potentially harmful foods and in quantities and proportions that are hazardous in a variety of ways including recommendations that will lead to disproportionate mineral absorption.

Cultural risk factors

Epidemiological data from third world nations shows a startling picture of iron deficiency in more than half the population of many of these countries. In some cases, this may be due to cultural practices in which animal products are not eaten, but this is likely only one contributor among many factors that compromise iron status in many poverty-ridden nations. Other dietary limitations, habits, choices and traditions are more likely to provide a more complete picture. As the burgeoning population of our planet presses us to harness all available food sources, we have reached a point where we are unable to sustain ourselves without inordinate consumption of grains (Cordain) and other relatively new foods.

Additional nutritional risk factors

Similarly, consumption of large quantities of dairy products is also likely to induce iron deficiency, especially in infants. This is likely the result of three interacting features of milk. These include dietary displacement of foods that can meet the our iron requirements, the presence of lactoferrin which binds to available iron in the intestine, perhaps compromising its absorption, and the very bio-available calcium in dairy products that competes with iron and other minerals for transport across the intestinal barrier. Thus, iron consumed in other foods may also be lost when consuming large quantities of cow's milk. It should not be surprising that infants who are fed cow's milk are reported as being at particularly high risk of developing iron deficiency (Bramhagen).

Similarly, adolescents' eating habits may also cause iron deficiency, particularly among females 11 to 18 years old followed by pubertal boys 11 to 14 years old (Thane).

These are stages of life associated with significant iron needs to support periods of rapid growth and, in the case of females, to compensate for iron losses during menses.

Based on the above data, several dietary factors can converge to confer iron deficiency. These include excessive milk and or whole grain consumption coupled with limited meat consumption.

Any individual who experiences chronic blood loss is also at an increased risk for iron deficiency. In addition to normal iron losses, the chronic bleeding would require inordinate iron consumption in order to forestall developing a deficiency. Such conditions that can induce an increased risk include celiac disease, where occult blood loss is the rule rather than the exception (Fine).

Food allergies and other intestinal diseases can also cause iron deficiency. Most dietary iron is absorbed in the proximal jejunum and the duodenum (Naveh). Diseases and allergies that cause damage in these regions of the small intestine are thus more likely to compromise absorption capacity resulting in iron malabsorption and consequent iron deficiency. Now let's look at how to improve our absorption of iron.

CHAPTER FOUR

Optimizing absorption

It is usually a mistake to maximize iron absorption at the expense of other minerals. Balanced absorption of all important minerals is a more appropriate goal than iron repletion at the cost of inadequate absorption of other minerals. Regular iron status testing will help in pursuit of this goal. For some of the same reasons that cow's milk consumption and/or large scale calcium supplementation is a poor nutritional strategy, excessive iron consumption and absorption is also problematic, and can even induce serious illness.

On the other hand, understanding some of the dynamics that control iron absorption will place you in a position to make the most of these processes when the need arises. As you have already seen, some of these strategies, such as whole grain and dairy product avoidance, drinking coffee, tea, wine, and cocoa at times well removed from mealtimes, and limiting or eliminating calcium supplements will benefit absorption of many valuable minerals including calcium, magnesium, copper, zinc, and, of course, iron. There is an unfortunate inclination, in some circles, to employ excessive measures, especially when it comes to supplementation, with the goal of rapid correction of the problem. This is a misguided approach that can be very dangerous. Time is a critical element in the restoration of iron sufficiency. Thus, employment of a complex of some of the carefully chosen dietary strategies outlined in this book, for optimizing absorption of o minerals, including iron, is the preferable course of action. Within the limited context of celiac patients, magnesium has been shown to benefit bone remineralization far more than calcium supplements (Rude) which suggests a compelling argument for a more balanced approach to ensuring mineral consumption. Thus the use of the above strategies holds the most promise for balanced absorption.

Heme and non-heme iron

Another step in this process is to ensure a general understanding of the differences between heme and non-heme iron, and how these differences can impact on absorption. About 40% of the iron from meats is in the form of heme iron which is quite easy to absorb. When easily absorbed, these minerals are said to be bioavailable. (Some claim that heme iron is absorbed at different intestinal receptors than other metals, but this issue is not yet well understood.) The other 60% of the iron in meats is non-heme iron which must be further processed in the gut. It is absorbed at intestinal receptors where other minerals are also absorbed. Foods derived from plants can only provide non-heme iron which is more difficult to absorb. (See table 2)

Table 2

Comparative absorption rates for heme and non-heme iron

Type of iron	Normal rates of absorption
heme	15% - 35%
non-heme	2% - 20%

Factors that aid iron absorption

Stomach acid

Stomach acids break down proteins, liberating the heme iron from the hemoglobin and myoglobin in meats we have consumed. These acids also liberate non-heme iron from the proteins to which it is bound. Vitamin C also contributes to liberating non-heme iron from compounds that are degraded by stomach acids, making iron available for absorption when it leaves the stomach. Most iron is absorbed across the intestinal barrier in that part of the intestine that is closest to the stomach, called the proximal duodenum. Thus, if iron is not freed in the stomach it is unlikely to be absorbed at all. (See figure 1)

Figure 1

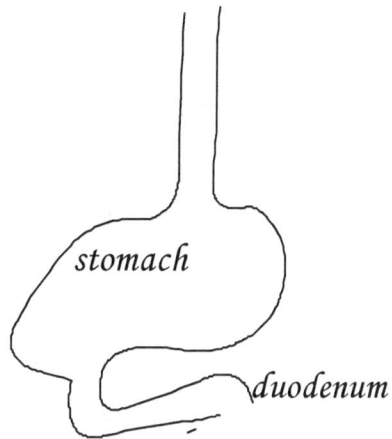

stomach

duodenum

Combining heme and non-heme iron

Some yet unknown, common factor in meat, fish, and poultry also enhances the absorption of non-heme iron.

It appears that meals that include both heme and non-heme iron result in increased absorption of both forms of iron. The addition of vitamin C further enhances absorption of non-heme iron.

Table 3

Dietary factors that enhance absorption of iron

Type of iron	Enhancers of absorption	
Heme iron	Reduced concurrent calcium intake; retention and food mixing in the stomach	
non-heme iron	pH level in the stomach (increased acidity improves absorption); ascorbic acid (can counteract the inhibitory impact of phytates and polyphenols); organic acids; animal tissues; Increased vitamin C intake at mealtime	

(data from Lynch, 1997)

A few sources of non-heme iron

Many foods are quite rich in non-heme iron. The following is a brief list of a few of the vegetables that contain large quantities of non-heme iron:

Bok choy   Peas

Figs	Black eye peas
Apricots	Pumpkin seeds
Sesame	Potato skins
Sunflower seeds	Beet greens
Cashews	Watercress
Dates	Brussels sprouts
Cooked broccoli	Raisins
Watermelon	

Heme iron

Meats, especially red meats, are rich in heme iron, so for optimal iron absorption, a meal that includes red meat and one or more of the above vegetables, preferably cooked, would be most beneficial in terms of iron absorption.

Supplements

Iron overload is often the result of supplementation in combination with a hereditary propensity to store excessive amounts of iron. This combination can lead to permanent damage to vital organs, and in extreme cases death is a possible consequence. Iron overload is a risk that accompanies excessive absorption and storage of iron.

On the other hand, those who experience iron deficiency, and are unable or unwilling to correct the matter through diet, may benefit from supplementation provided regular testing of hemoglobin and iron stores is undertaken and these test results are carefully monitored.

Oral iron is the most common and most benign approach. Constipation and stomach upset are the most severe side effects. Of course, if inadequate intestinal absorption of iron is the underlying cause of the iron deficiency, such supplements are likely to cause these unpleasant side effects without providing a remedy for the iron deficiency. Intravenous iron injections, on the other hand, may not be so benign, but they circumvent the problems that are often associated with absorbing oral iron supplements. The concerns that have been raised about intravenous iron include an increased risk of infection, anaphylaxis, oxidative stress, and cardiovascular disease (Cavill).

When readers optimize their iron status it is unlikely to cause sudden, dramatic changes in intellectual capacities and learning potentials. Six weeks is the minimum delay before any measurable change can be seen, and most studies suggest that a longer delay is probable. A more likely result of improved iron status is a complex of many small improvements in memory, performance, and wellness that are so gradual in their onset that they will be missed by all but the most astute observers.

Still, it is clear that iron repletion or iron sufficiency is a very legitimate goal for a variety of reasons including improved health, cognition, and memory. As mentioned at the beginning of this chapter, iron repletion should be sought only in concert with optimizing absorption of all important minerals. Excessive iron intake and absorption may interfere with calcium, magnesium, zinc, and copper status, with all the health problems associated with these critical minerals, including muscle action, bone density, immune function, etc. A thoughtful, balanced approach will ensure adequate, appropriate absorption of all of these minerals and, other factors being equal, the robust good health that usually ensues in this context. In the next chapter we will look more closely at just how iron has all of these myriad impacts on the human body and brain.

CHAPTER FIVE

Some basics of iron metabolism

Iron is an essential nutrient. Without it we could not live. Iron is involved in the synthesis of hemoglobin. It participates in energy conversion at the cellular level, and is a factor in the synthesis of neurotransmitters and enzymes. Recent investigations also suggest that iron is important to several processes directly related to brain function. These include iron's involvement in myelin formation, the function of the hippocampus, and in modulating insulin sensitivity. Some of these biological functions of iron change as we move from one stage of life to the next. Thus, differences in iron metabolism as it relates to the general life stages of childhood, adulthood, and senior adulthood are also important.

Synthesis of hemoglobin and its function

Transferrin is the protein that transports iron to the bone marrow where it is used to produce red blood cells. Hemoglobin contributes one third of the weight of red blood cells. These hemoglobin cells begin in bone marrow. They move through several developmental stages before they reach the point where they synthesize the internal protein hemoglobin. Each red blood cell destined to become hemoglobin will move through several more stages during which it loses its nucleus and other cellular features while it develops its unique circular form, with two concave sides. The large surface area of the two concave sides allows easy attachment of iron and which is ideal for the transfer of oxygen and, to a lesser extent, carbon dioxide.

It is the appropriate absorption, distribution, and release of these two gases that form this cell's primary function throughout its survival of about one hundred and twenty days. Hemoglobin is responsible for all of the body's oxygen distribution requirements, and about one quarter of its carbon dioxide transportation and expulsion through the lungs.

The portion of carbon dioxide transportation that is handled by hemoglobin is partly the result of the binding and release of carbon dioxide by the amino acids in the globin portion of hemoglobin proteins and hence is of only tangential relevance to our interests here.

The iron portion of hemoglobin binds to oxygen. Hemoglobin is the oxygen carrying protein that gives whole blood its red color. A hemoglobin molecule is made up of a protein called globin combined with four non protein pigments called hemes. Each heme contains an iron ion that can combine reversibly with one oxygen molecule, and each red blood cell contains about 280 million hemoglobin molecules. As blood passes the lung membranes, oxygen moves through that membrane, enters red blood cells, and combines with the iron ion components of hemoglobin to form oxyhemoglobin. In this form, red blood cells circulate to various tissues and organs throughout the body, releasing the oxygen into surrounding fluids to meet the oxygen needs of nearby cells.

Because it is so critical to human survival, the oxygen distribution function of the iron portion of hemoglobin is clearly necessary to learning. Without oxygen, the brain cells can neither encode memories nor survive. Few would argue against the proposition that learning can be compromised by reduced oxygen supply to the brain in the context of iron deficiency anemia.

However, such a state of anemia is at the extreme end of the iron deficiency continuum. The primary debate that is ongoing within the medical literature about the significance of iron stores in the learning process is somewhat apart from the frank, widespread admission that iron deficiency anemia can not help but compromise the learning capacities, memory, and coordination of the individual so afflicted, and this negative impact goes far beyond the limiting potentials listed here.

ATP synthesis, muscles and energy conversion

Iron is also involved in many other bodily processes and functions. Ferritin, the protein that stores iron, is found in almost all cells of the body. Although most ferritin is found in the liver and the spleen, the biological importance of iron is implied by the widespread presence of these iron storage proteins.

In keeping with the sliding filament theory, each muscle movement requires many molecules of adenosine triphosphate (ATP) at each of the many binding sites on the myosin cross-bridges of each muscle fiber. As the energy source for muscle contraction, ATP works in conjunction with calcium ions to shorten, or attempt to shorten, muscle length. ATP also provides energy for other cellular functions in the body, including reactions that build body tissues as well as the task of moving substances in or out of cells.

A typical cell contains about a billion molecules of ATP, and the enzymes involved in the synthesis of each ATP molecule requires iron for its own synthesis. Thus, a pre-requisite of each tiny muscle movement is the widespread presence of iron stores throughout the body.

Iron's importance to neurotransmitter synthesis and function

Similarly, many millions of nerve axons thread throughout our bodies, including our brains, permitting the coordinated communication that we rely on for mobility, organ function, and survival. Each of the billions of connections between these nerves, called synapses, requires a compliment of neurotransmitters to effectively relay the messages from one axon to the next. Iron plays a pivotal role in this venue of our physiology through its contribution as a cofactor in the synthesis and function of several important neurotransmitters.

Dopamine, noradrenaline, and serotonin are among those neurotransmitters that require iron for their synthesis. These neurotransmitters are also important to a variety of processes and psychological states. Dopamine is not only involved in movement, it is also involved in both attention and learning. Not only is iron involved in the synthesis of acetylcholine (Swartz-Basile) this neurotransmitter is also involved in several brain functions related to learning, particularly in relation to memory and coordination which are encoded in a process that involves the hippocampus and the striatum (Rogers) (Ragozzino). Some evidence also suggests that iron is involved in anticipation and planning (Dagher). Iron is a pivotal component in the formation of long-term memories in the hippocampus. This portion of the brain is thus the location of the first event in a process that leads to the storage of more permanent memories.

The hippocampus is thought to process declarative memories then export them for storage in the outer layer of the brain called the cerebral cortex. Once memories are formed, the hippocampus is not needed for retrieval of these memories. It can go on encoding current experiences into memories. However, since the hippocampus is a major repository of brain iron, it appears that iron is of critical importance to hippocampal function. During periods of low iron stores, hippocampal function is impeded. Thus, absent mindedness may be more of a reflection of iron deficiency than of preoccupation with more important matters.

Iron's involvement in myelin formation

Iron also aids in the formation of myelin, a fatty substance that improves the conductivity of nerves through insulating the nerve axons from exterior ionic and chemical interference. The recent discovery of this function of iron provides a framework for understanding the impact of anemia during critical growth stages of infancy. Developmental delays and apparently permanent states of mild to moderate mental retardation may be the result of delayed synthesis of myelin for the central nervous system (Hurtado).

Iron deficiency can alter mood and insulin sensitivity

Even iron deficiency isn't all bad. Iron deficiency can also impact on our behavior indirectly through its impact on our ability to metabolize glucose. This is one apparent benefit of iron deficiency which may involve a lower risk of developing diabetes (Hua, Stoohs, Facchini). (Conversely, iron overload can increase the risk of insulin resistance and type 2 diabetes.)

Iron deficiency without anemia is an area in which there are many disparate perspectives and a wide range of

46

research results. Everyone, it seems, has a different opinion. Nonetheless, a careful examination of the data suggests that iron deficiency may be a very major player in many learning and behavioral problems among school children as well as limiting quality of life for many children and adults.

In the next chapter we will look at how all this impacts on learning.

CHAPTER SIX

Iron status and learning

All of the roles outlined in the previous chapter for iron in neurological/brain maintenance offer insights into the many findings relating iron deficiency to learning, memory, and other cognitive deficits.

Iron deficiency and the brain

The brain is just one location where the negative impact of reduced oxygen supply to any part of the body, especially the brain, is a very reasonable cause for concern. However, such hemoglobin related issues are of greater concern in more advanced cases of iron deficiency where advanced anemia is either present or imminent. These latter are usually preceded by deficiencies in iron stores which can be identified by measuring the presence of ferritin, an iron storage protein, and transferrin, an iron transport protein.

Investigations of the impact of iron deficiency on school performance suggest that it is a more complex issue than simply iron's contribution to the oxygen distribution. Many researchers report that learning inhibition occurs long before the reduced hemoglobin of iron deficiency anemia develops (Zlotkin)(Halterman)(Yehuda).

The controversies that surround iron status and learning are grounded in considerable evidence on all sides. One group presents iron supplementation as an exciting new educational tool, demonstrating that scores on standardized Mathematics examinations and in some domains of I.Q. testing are significantly affected by the iron status of high school students. According to others, the potential learning gains, as indicated by the differences in achievement according to iron status, may not warrant the enthusiasm with which they are sometimes endorsed. The critics of the studies showing improved learning from iron supplements are dismissive, characterizing the results as minor, and arguing that iron supplements offer relatively little change in student learning and achievement. Conversely, peer reviewed research publications in the field of brain function clearly show that iron is an integral part of the process by which the hippocampus encodes long-term memory. Thus, studies of iron supplementation over very short periods, may only hint at the dramatic learning and achievement possibilities offered by life-long iron sufficiency.

Three theories about how iron causes cognitive problems

Yehuda and Rabinovitz have outlined three current theories that have been offered to explain why iron deficiency can result in cognitive deficits. The first is based on the observed disruption of normal sleep-wake patterns (called circadian rhythms) and disruption of consistent body temperatures (called thermoregulation) caused by iron deficiency. This theory postulates that such changes in body rhythm and regulation will lead to altered test performance.

The second theory points to the reduced dopamine levels caused by iron deficiency. Recognition of the important and extensive role that dopamine plays in several forms of learning, suggests that iron deficiency may inhibit learning through reducing dopamine levels.

The third theory is rooted in the role of the hippocampus in encoding long term memories. An important facet of this theory is the increased vulnerability of the hippocampus during iron deficiency. After stress or injury, this memory gateway is less likely to perform well if there was a concurrent state of iron deficiency. This latter theory harkens to the association between damage to the hippocampus and cognitive deficits especially as seen in Alzheimer's and other forms of dementia.

Perhaps an amalgam of the above theories may offer the most valid insights into this issue.

Some element of this may also be due to one or more of the many other functions iron serves within the brain. For instance. Neuotransmitters are critical components in communication between cells and regions within the brain. Drastic reduction of dopamine, a neurotransmitter that is involved in many facets of behavior, has been shown in animal studies to occur in association with iron deficiency. Similar studies have also shown that iron deficiency can compromise the integrity of the blood brain barrier, which normally protects the brain from a host of hazards (often of dietary origins) that can gain access to the bloodstream and would not normally be allowed to access the brain.

As mentioned in the previous chapter, iron helps us to encode long term memory. Any memory that lasts more than a few minutes is usually a long-term memory. Such memories are thought to be consolidated during our sleep, but the hippocampus has long been recognized as being a critical link in the memory encoding process. The hippocampus has been characterized as the gateway to memory (Wolfe) and the gates are made of iron.

Iron has also been identified as a cofactor in the myelinization of nerve axons (Lozoff). Myelin is the substance that surrounds, protects, and insulates nerve tissues, allowing high speed transmission of electrical nerve impulses. Without myelin, these electrical impulses will be lost or weakened through dissipation into surrounding tissues. Just as the electrical wiring in your house must be insulated to restrict the electrical charge to its intended path, nerves often require myelin to restrict the electrical signals to the nerve axons.

Iron is also involved in enzyme metabolism related to muscle cell activity (through a substance called adenosine tri-phosphate), ion transport, protein synthesis, and iron storage in various regions of the brain and body.

Iron deficient infants

For thirty years one group of iron deficient infants and children was studied to see what happens to them as they grow and mature (Oski). The results clearly show improved mental acuity, as measured by a wide range of tests, after iron repletion. However, it is also equally clear that correction of the problem is nowhere near as effective in improving intellectual performance as avoiding the problem before it gets a start.

According to Yehuda and Rabinovitz, the duration and the magnitude of iron deficiency "determine the degree of cognitive deficit" that will result. It is thus of vital importance that expectant mothers ensure a healthy iron status for themselves during pregnancy and lactation, as well as for their children as they grow and develop.

Menstruation, Mathematics, and iron

Gender can have a significant impact on iron status. The onset of menstruation appears to coincide with reduced performance in Mathematics among many girls/young women . Two studies have mapped the performance of secondary female students in the field of Mathematics (Halterman) and I.Q. testing (Bruner) and have shown a significant relationship between iron deficiency and compromised performance in the first study, and improved performance resulting from iron supplementation.

Iron is clearly of some importance in the learning process. Since a large segment of the population suffers from iron deficiency in the absence of anemia, this deficiency can also be shown to lead to some very serious learning consequences. Our cultural failure to monitor and correct iron deficiencies causes a serious loss of educational and productive capacities that can be extremely costly.

My classroom experience

I am proud to have spent the last several years of my teaching career working at a school where we went to great lengths to provide pregnant teens with full access to educational opportunities. During that time I observed a phenomenon that many of my colleagues called "baby brain." During their final months, many of these students would easily become confused and were often forgetful.

I realize that the anecdotal experiences, as reflected above on are not as credible as the results of a carefully controlled study. They are simply my observations of factors that I can not even definitely identify or quantify. After all, I have not observed students taking supplements or following any other protocol for improving their iron status. I am simply trusting what students have told me about such matters and trusting my memory as much of these comments were never written down. Nonetheless, each student has contributed to the personal, practical knowledge that I have accumulated during my twenty years in the classroom observing children while they learned and grew.

Because I have been interested in iron metabolism for some time, I have often spoken to students and/or their parents about my concerns. When asked about the student's iron status – whether it has been checked recently and if so, what the results indicated, I have been given a variety of responses. Sometimes my concerns were completely ill founded. Recent testing or some other information clearly established that I was wrong to be concerned. More often my concerns were well founded. Some students acknowledged that they had anemia. Others indicated they had not been tested. Some had never, to their knowledge, been tested Still others informed me that since I am not a medical doctor I should mind my own business. In the latter cases, I simply abandoned the issue. For the most part, parents and students were grateful for my interest and suggestions. Only once did I hear back that a physician had refused to test a student's iron status based on my suggestion. In most other cases the students were tested. My suspicions were frequently correct and hence, proved a valuable contribution to students' wellness and school performance.

How students respond to iron supplements

It is my experience that when iron deficient students started on iron supplements or undertook to improve their iron status by dietary means, they soon became better readers. Although I did not notice any change in reading speed, there was a consistent trend of improvement in comprehension which was usually reflected in improved reading test scores or improved performance on assignments based on their reading. These students also seemed more alert and more attentive during class.

Some of the controversies

Iron deficiency anemia is widely accepted as a cause of learning problems. This is not in dispute. In combination with the widespread recognition of memory disturbances as a symptom of deficient iron stores, this makes it difficult to deny that iron deficiency can, and frequently does, impact on learning.

The important question is really one of how seriously to take this issue. For instance, are relatively mild states of anemia, or relatively mild cases of depleted iron stores important to health and/or learning issues? Can and do they alter learning capacities significantly and in ways that should be of interest or concern to readers?

For instance, is the ability to encode short or long-term memories compromised when non-anemic students simply do not have sufficient iron stores? Are our reflexes dampened or altered? Is our ability to focus and maintain attention compromised by low iron stores? Are we more motivated or more active learners the more closely we approach iron repletion? What implications does iron status have for our curiosity and our thirst for knowledge? What impact does a state of low iron stores, and its subsequent influence over the synthesis of various neurotransmitters, have on one's ability behave and make the most of educational opportunities? I believe that the answer to all of the above questions is yes but not everyone agrees.

Despite this widespread acceptance of anemia as deleterious to learning, several meta-analysis investigations reveal that confounding factors such as socio-economic conditions have not been effectively isolated and excluded as contributing factors in many of the studies reporting an association between iron deficiencies and compromised learning capacities (Grantham-McGregor, Ani, 2001). The same researchers also express concerns about whether iron supplementation intervention will reverse the negative impact of iron deficiency anemia. They examined eight studies of non-anemic, iron deficient subjects in which there is considerable variation in baseline findings between control and experimental groups, I.Q. or performance testing methods, and the types of learning capacities being measured. Not surprisingly, their findings are also widely disparate. Some report significant improvements in the children's learning capacities (or their attentional focus and motivation) while others found no significant improvements in school achievements. Notably, even among those studies reporting improvements, only one study reported subjects, in only one test domain, as recovering to the level of iron-replete controls (Grantham-McGregor).

Others, conducting another meta-analysis, reported that short-term iron supplementation (5 to 11 days) does not have a discernible effect on psycho motor development, but interventions lasting from 30 days to 4 months do show a positive, significant impact of iron supplementation on psycho motor development among anemic children (Logan).

Individuals with low iron stores are widespread and numerous. It is a condition that is altered by a variety of factors. While most researchers are reporting some degree of cognitive and psycho motor improvement following iron supplementation, there is still some disagreement about the impact on learning capacities. There is also debate about specific types of testing employed to identify improvements (or the absence thereof) in learning. Some are examining vocabulary development, short-term memory, others examine long-term memory, yet others test for improvements in attention span, psycho motor development, or various linguistic competencies.

I have already mentioned the widespread distribution and function of iron within the body, from muscle action and coordination, to neurotransmission, to brain function, and sugar metabolism. Each of these factors has been shown elsewhere to act as mediators of learning (Santucci) (Timmann)(Suh). Further, each of these elements may, to some extent, interact. For instance, well coordinated muscle action increases the likelihood of participation in sports and other activities, which improves circulation, carrying and distributing nutrients throughout the entire body, including the brain.

Also, neurotransmission is not only necessary for muscle activation and sensing our environments, it contributes to our mental and emotional states including our senses of well-being and security, all of which are well established elements in the learning process. For instance, depressed individuals may not be as interested in learning. Glucose metabolism is yet another element of human physiology that has repeatedly been shown to impact on mood, behavior, and learning.

Some incomplete answers

Several other reports show improved learning capacities, among iron deficient individuals following iron supplementation. For instance, one literature review indicates that children over the age of three years are more likely to benefit from iron supplementation in the identified domains of "achievement at school, concentration, discriminant learning, short term memory, and IQ." (Pettifor). The same report explains forms of mild to moderate iron deficiency, in the absence of anemia, in which tissue function is impaired, particularly in areas related to learning. The same authors explore the well documented association between cases of iron deficiency and "impaired development in behavior, cognition, and psycho motor skills". Pettifor goes on to discuss eight double blind trials, six of which report improvements in students' learning in one or more of a range of domains as measured by a variety of instruments.

Significantly, one of these studies found improved psychomotor and language development after one year of iron supplementation. It also showed that improvements in language development occur as the indirect result of iron supplementation on factors other than hemoglobin levels (Stoltzfus). This was revealed through the limited impact of iron supplementation on the hemoglobin levels in all but the most anemic subjects in this investigation. This illuminating but anomalous response to supplementation was likely due to the widespread presence of parasitic worms in the study population. Importantly, 97% of these pre-school subjects were anemic by international standards. These investigators also found widespread malaria among their subjects, which increased the complexity of their findings. These compounding factors aided in isolating the correlation between improved language development and improved iron status exclusive of hemoglobin levels.

Further evidence in support of iron supplementation, toward improved iron stores, and leading to improved learning is found in an investigation of a group of non-anemic, iron deficient, female high school students in Baltimore, Maryland. The experimental group achieved significant improvements in recall performance when compared with their baseline performance at the beginning of the trial. Of at least equal importance, the control group did not show similar improvement (Bruner). It is important to recognize that this study was conducted with subjects whose iron deficiency was in iron stores alone. Subjects who developed anemia were dropped from the study and their anemia was treated.

While critics point to the three measures of attention in which these students did not show significant improvement (Walker & Walker) this report of improved recall may be of great interest to readers and anyone else who is interested in improving their memory through optimizing their iron status.

Yet another perspective seeks to harness the education system to help remediate the growing problem of iron deficiency. An opposing view holds that education funding should be diverted to iron supplementation programs that provide children with adequate iron supplementation. It does seem reasonable to assert that children's health must be taken care of before education becomes a consideration. However, it is also arguable that children may benefit more from learning the importance and available sources of dietary iron.

As has been demonstrated by decades of foreign aid programs, self-sufficiency is less likely to develop through the simple provision and distribution of supplements. If, on the other hand, education is seen as the facilitation of increasing levels of independence, then harnessing the education system toward increased awareness and positive action for improving students' iron status is the preferable alternative. Nonetheless, there is merit to both sides of the argument. In an ideal world adequate funding would be provided to both education and iron supplementation programs.

Harnessing the controversies

We do not have all the relevant information, and the range of divergent opinions threatens to obscure important answers. On the other hand, these various perspectives may also be used to paint a clearer picture of the impact of iron deficiency on learning. On the whole, the evidence indicates that iron deficiency both with and without anemia is deleterious to learning. Further, compromised learning usually appears long before iron deficiency reaches the stage of anemia.

We know that iron is a necessary component in a wide range of activities within the body and brain. We also know that many of these functions are critical to various elements of learning. As for the studies that appear to negate the value of intervention, usually in the form of supplements, any of a number of intervening factors may have served to reduce their value, including poor absorption, dietary co-factors, intestinal infections, or excessive blood loss. Any one or more of these possibilities would serve to mitigate the results reported. Similarly, the testing employed by the two groups who reported no significant improvements may not be sufficiently sensitive to identify improvement. The duration of the trials may also have been too short. As was noted earlier, short trials of iron supplementation typically do not result in measurable improvements in learning. It is also quite possible that supplementation simply may not always be a viable answer to iron deficiency.

However, there are several ways to achieve iron repletion. Oral supplements may be among the poorest of these alternatives. This is where the lifestyle choices and dietary practices, as outlined previously, may be helpful. On the other hand, supplements may be the only reasonable option in some circumstances.

CHAPTER SEVEN

Tests to request and interpreting them

Each preceding chapter has offered evidence, anecdotes, and information building toward a cohesive view of iron metabolism, how deficiencies arise, and appropriate strategies for correction and/or maintenance of iron status, as suggested by test results. We have now arrived at the very heart of this book's message. Testing is a critical component of a thoughtful, healthy approach to managing one's iron status. Interpretation of test results and appropriate follow-up strategies for normalizing or maintaining healthy iron status are the next steps in this process.

The scientific community's understanding of iron metabolism is incomplete. Despite some differing views, authorities agree that certain biological imperatives dictate our need for significant quantities of iron on a regular basis.

Table 4 lists several different blood components that will reflect one or more features of iron status. For instance, low platelet counts can signify a condition of low iron. More direct measures of iron status include hematocrit, which measures the quantities of red blood cells as a percentage of total blood. These red cells are called erythrocytes and they provide a structure to hold hemoglobin. Transferrin is a protein that transports iron, and ferritin is an iron storage protein.

Table 4

Measurements of the various forms of iron in the body

Blood component	Normal range	Units of measurement
Hematocrit	Male 40-54	% of blood by volume
	Female 38-46	% of blood by volume
Platelet count	140-450x10³	Per microliter
Transferrin	204-360	mg/Dl
Ferritin	18-250 male	ng/mL
	12-160 female	ng/mL

data from Tortora & Grabowski, 1996)

Important information may be gleaned from test reports simply through understanding some of the standard abbreviations that are used in the reports. For instance, although hematocrit (Hct) test results are sometimes given as raw numbers, the number actually represents the volume of red blood cells compared to the total volume of blood, in the form of a percentage value. Thus, an Hct of 45 would indicate that 45% of the blood volume was made up of red blood cells. The normal range for Hct is 38-46 in adult females and 40-54 in adult males. Hct testing is one of those venues where a patient's awareness of prior test results can be very revealing. For instance, "A significant drop in hematocrit indicates anemia." (Tortora and Grabowski)

Hemoglobin, the iron-containing protein that forms part of the red blood cell, is measured in grams per hundred millilitres of blood, with normal values for infants and adults given in Table 5. The "reference range" outlines the values that are considered normal. Thus, results that fall outside the reference range would be considered abnormal.

Table 5

Normal values for hemoglobin

Stage of life & gender	Low	High	
Infants	Below 14	Above 20	grams/100ml of blood
Adult females	Below 12	Above 16	grams/100ml of blood
Adult males	Below 13.5	Above 18	grams/100ml of blood

(developed from data from Tortora and Grabowski, 1996)

Transferrin is a plasma protein that transports two iron ions in the bloodstream until it encounters a cell that shows a transferrin receptor on its surface. Through a process of absorption and subsequent release of the transferrin after chemically extracting the iron, the transferrin is now free to circulate and attach more iron ions. The normal range for transferrin is 22-45 micromoles per litter of blood.

Apoferritin is a protein that can store iron. When it combines with the iron it stores, it forms ferritin. Each ferritin molecule can store up to approximately 4,500 atoms of iron. Thus, ferritin is measured by determining the quantity of iron, in monograms, per millilitre of serum. The normal range is 18-250 ng/ml of serum in males and 12-160 ng/ml of serum in females. Testing for ferritin saturation is, according to many investigators, the test of choice for identifying mild to moderate cases of hemochromatosis, or iron overload (Herbert). When ferritin levels rise above the reference range, iron overload is extremely likely and a physician should be consulted. .

Turn to the next chapter to see just who not to take dietary advice from.

CHAPTER EIGHT

Relevant nutritional controversies

Whose dietary advice can we trust?

Some scientists are attacking the USDA's food guide. Each criticism is based on one or more of several complaints. Some investigators assert that the food guide pyramid reflects a conflict of interests on the part of the USDA (Braly and Hoggan, 2002) (Willett, 2002). Others have pointed to the undue influence exerted by special interest groups such as dairy councils & grain producers in contesting some elements while shaping others in their own economic interests (Nestle, 1993). Neither does this guide address the needs of illness groups where diet is the treatment of choice (Braly and Hoggan, 2002). Also, compliance with the recommendations of the food guide provides little protection from major and chronic diseases. Thus, the healthy eating index is only slightly healthier than the average American's approach to eating (McCullough). Many current scientific studies refute, in one way or another, most of the underlying beliefs on which the healthy eating guide is based. Given such data, it should not be surprising to find that there is considerable evidence that political and economic interests are involved in shaping these food guides and their recommendations (Nestle, 1993).

How do these recommendations impact on iron status?

Even a cursory glance at any of the many editions of the USDA food guide published over the last century reveals that grains, particularly whole grains, are recommended for frequent, large-scale, daily consumption.

Evidence presented in earlier chapters shows that following these recommendations is likely to inhibit absorption of iron and other important minerals.

Another important facet of USDA food recommendations is their advocacy of dairy products. These foods are often, and with good cause, touted for their significant calcium content which is in a highly bio-available form. Lactoferrin, a component of the whey fraction of cow's milk has an iron binding capacity that is 260 times greater than transferrin. This feature, in combination with the impact of calcium and the very low levels of iron found in dairy products, further threaten the iron sufficiency of those who follow the recommendations of this eating guide.

Should the food pyramid be changed?

Many critics would argue for adjusting the USDA's food guide, but such a simple expedient may not be as easily accomplished as we might first expect. The same political and economic forces that have helped shape these recommendations are unlikely to surrender profits and market shares because of the epidemiological data related to iron sufficiency. Neither are politicians likely to forego votes, and campaign contributions on the same basis. Such scenarios are particularly unlikely in view of the predictable consequences of such adjustments to the food guide.

Changes to the USDA's recommendations for healthy eating would also relegate improved health only to those who can afford less abundant, increasingly sought-after foods. Changes to the food guide may need to follow changes in marketplace demands, which is more likely to result in more gradual and stable changes to our food supply. By this I mean that there are many books entering and newly on the market that debunk government food guides. They may have a combined impact of causing a gradual shift in public dietary habits and choices. Such gradual changes in demand will drive similar changes in supply, ultimately changing conventional wisdom. Conversely, dramatic changes might cause a seriously destabilizing impact that would compromise both current food production and new food production systems aimed at improved nutrition through responding to scientific evidence regarding optimal human nutrition.

CHAPTER NINE

Iron Overload

My first manuscript did not include a discussion of iron overload. This is partly because my knowledge is limited in this area. Still, it seemed irresponsible not to offer at least a very basic explanation of this condition, as it can pose a serious hazard to some people. This is especially true for those who have had a recent diagnosis of some intestinal or other ailment that causes chronic blood-loss. It is also true for anyone who goes ahead with the iron management strategies included here without first getting appropriate blood tests. The deciding factor in the decision to include this information was recalling an acquaintance whose story you will read shortly.

What is iron overload?

Iron overload results from the absorption of too much iron. In developed nations, it is usually the result of a recessive gene. That means that it must have come from both parents. Although it is commonly thought of as a genetic defect, this trait may have conferred some survival advantage, especially in situations where meat is scarce.

The problem doesn't manifest until adulthood, when the iron needs for growth outstrip supply, even among those with a genetic inclination to store too much iron. It is after adulthood is reached, and in the absence of other iron losses that iron stores begin to rise. The rate of rise will depend on a number of factors including iron supplements and iron consumption. Regular blood donation, involvement in rigorous sports, and illnesses such as celiac disease will often slow the rate of iron storage. The net result is that symptoms may arise early in adulthood, or decades later.

Due to menstruation, women with overload will be slower to manifest symptoms and onset may be delayed for many years. The best way to detect iron overload, or hemochromatosis, is by checking the blood for ferritin levels and transferrin saturation, which should be at or below 44%.

Symptoms of overload

This is particularly important in cases of recently diagnosed illnesses, such as celiac disease, where the cause of blood loss is corrected by treatment of the celiac disease so iron stores will begin to build. I know a man who was in just this situation. He felt that he had found the answer to his health problems with his celiac diagnosis. He felt well on the gluten free diet for some time. Then his health began to decline.

At first he thought traces of gluten must have been getting into his diet from somewhere. He went through a slow process of testing for a variety of ailments. He had some difficulty with his health insurance. He had to leave university and go to work to meet the escalating costs of his medical care, and the delays due to these mounting costs further delayed the diagnostic process.

What had started as a general feeling of malaise with low energy levels and a sense of fatigue soon degraded into much more serious symptoms. He began to doubt his own sanity as he struggled with severe, recurring stomach pains and joint pains for which there was no apparent cost. He lost a tremendous amount of weight.

As an individual's iron stores increase, they experience a loss of sex drive, they begin to lose pubic hair, they may experience shortness of breath, and women may stop menstruating or experience early menopause.

Diagnosing iron overload

Finally, someone noticed his increased ferritin levels and wondered if that might indicate the cause of his symptoms. When last we spoke, about ten years ago in North Carolina, he did not know if or how much his vital organs had been damaged. I have since lost touch with him, and would welcome hearing from him again, as I wonder about how he has fared.

His story should alert readers to the need for iron testing, even if they do nothing else to manage their iron metabolism, it is important to be vigilant about the risk of iron overload, or hemochromatosis as it is called by the medical profession.

Advanced cases of overload

In advanced of cases of iron overload, excessive iron is stored in the liver, where it can cause cirrhosis and/or liver cancer. It can also cause arthritis, high blood sugar, insulin resistance, and chronic stomach pains. There are two common skin discolorations that often arise in the context of advanced iron overload. One is a grey pallor, and the other is a bronze/yellowish color.

In researching the materials for this chapter, I suddenly realized that someone close to me might well have iron overload. After contacting him and asking about recent blood test results, my suspicions are running very high. I have been working with him on a diet to control his insulin resistance, and I now realize that the insulin resistance and a very recent onset of arthritic pain may be the result of his excessive iron stores, although he also shows signs of mild anemia. This is very exciting news, as I now suspect that a rapid improvement in all of his symptoms may soon be in the offing.

CHAPTER TEN

Summary

If we are to stem the tide of iron deficiency that is currently sweeping the world, we must take bold steps. It is imperative that we learn enough about our iron needs to ensure our own health and that of our children. If we can be moved to take responsibility for managing our iron status and to take steps to maintain healthy levels of iron stores and hemoglobin, we and our children will benefit. Our next step is to share this information with the world. Such knowledge will lead to improved parental feeding practices, and the cycle of remediation will have begun.

Further research is needed

Despite the controversies, there can be little doubt that iron status does impact our memory, learning capacities and general wellness. The study that manipulated the iron status of selected students their deficiencies were mild and showed improvements on I.Q. testing after a brief period of iron supplementation (Bruner). Another study compared students' iron status and their performance on Mathematics exams and found that iron deficiency predicted lower performance (Halterman). In yet another study, motor and language development were shown to improve following iron supplementation (Stoltzfus). Conversely, iron deficiency during infancy has been shown to cause more severe and long-lasting consequences. Similarly, iron overload can be an important factor in some psychiatric illnesses (Cutler) and a host of mild to deadly symptoms and associated illnesses. Clearly, iron status can affect the function of the brain. The controversies highlight the importance of a conservative and cautious approach to managing iron status, including regular testing, appropriate diet and food preparation, aimed at ensuring optimal iron status.

The areas of disagreement also highlight the need for much more study of this medically and educationally important issue. For instance, it would be valuable to have a clearer sense of the extent and nature of improvements we might encounter in the learning capacities of anemic and iron deficient individuals as their iron status approaches the reference range. It would also be useful to know more about adults and seniors; especially regarding just how long it takes for them to recover full intellectual function and at exactly what stage this occurs in their movement toward iron repletion as well as the extent of improvement that will result from normalizing their iron status.

Of course, this book is limited by the quality of the publications that informed it as well as our current, limited understandings of the iron needs and iron-mediated functions of the brain, along with the author's limitations in interpreting these data.

The peer review process

As most of the data reported here are drawn from the peer reviewed literature, it may be useful to examine exactly what that means. The peer review process requires that a paper submitted for publication is examined by a group of reviewers who are experts in the area that the article discusses. Most peer reviewed journals want to publish research results based on double blind cross-over studies. This research format is very expensive, time-consuming, and often impracticable, thus considerably narrowing the number of prospective articles. Experts in any field have built a reputation on their own achievements. They will have a vested interest in the furtherance of their own ideas and ones that are compatible with their own work. This causes considerable resistance to new ideas, especially if those new ideas pose a threat to the reviewer's work and/or professional prestige. The net result is that peer reviewed medical literature is extremely conservative. When, in the context of this literature we read comments to the effect that there is a current "epidemic" of iron deficiency, this is not likely to be a radical fringe perspective.

We will learn more as the scientific community advances into the vast areas of mystery that surround iron sufficiency and its impacts on brain function. In the interim, the safest course appears to be one of encouraging learning to monitor our own iron status and to become our own advocates on such important health issues.

Patient self-management

Patient self-management is already the norm in the context of many conditions such as diabetes, where patients are expected to monitor and regulate their blood sugar levels through a combination of insulin and diet (Lombardo). Self-monitoring and drug administration is also the largest component of standard treatments for other ailments such as asthma (Wolf)

Thus, patient self-management of iron status is not a large departure from current standards of practice employed with other conditions where nutrition may play an important role. Because iron deficiency is present in epidemic proportions, even in the affluent, industrialized nations, broad, school-based programs that educate students about these concerns may reduce the burden on our increasingly challenged health care system. Regular laboratory testing and individual self-assessment and management of iron status could be extremely beneficial in most cases. Where iron deficiency is signaling the presence of an underlying disease, supplements and dietary intervention will have little or no impact and a physician should be consulted.

Education

If the purpose of education is to increase student independence within a given domain, then an iron sufficiency program offers considerable promise. Not only does it offer to increase the independence of students regarding their iron status, it also offers to make them better consumers of health care services, and heighten their awareness of nutrition as a science in its infancy. Broad education in the field of the germ theory, beginning early in the 20th Century followed and accompanied the widespread acceptance of the germ theory paradigm within the scientific community of that epoch. School children were suddenly cast into a world where they could observe and predict the behavior of microscopic organisms that were once characterized as "invisible atomies".

Similarly, today's citizens of democracy can participate in the unfolding of the 21st Century's embrace of nutritional controversies, ailments, and paradigms. The social construction of the field of nutritoxicity is under way. We can prepare students with the independence, knowledge, skills, and attributes to critically examine and select the information based on evidence. More than one researcher has gone on record recommending school-based instruction of iron metabolism and supplementation. The widespread ignorance of this dietary issue ensues and is perpetuated if we fail to take action to reverse the unfortunate trend that has been characterized as an epidemic.

More knowledgeable students will become adults and parents who will make wiser choices for themselves, their children, and their loved ones. And the healing will have begun.

Let's stay in touch.

Contact me at:

hoggan@shaw.ca

Or go to:

http://www.ironedge.info

to stay up to date on iron metabolism

(Anticipated website upload date: June, 2008)

GLOSSARY:

Iron therapy. Iron therapy is defined as the prescription and subsequent injection or oral ingestion of iron in pill, liquid, or other form, by a qualified health care professional.

Iron deficiency anemia. Iron deficiency anemia is defined as reduced levels of hemoglobin, a blood protein, formed partly from iron, which assimilates, transports, and distributes oxygen.

Iron deficiency. Iron deficiency is defined as less than 12 grams per liter (μg/L) of blood in adults, and less than 14 μg/L of blood in children

Ferritin is defined as "The major iron storage protein. The blood level of ferritin serves as an indicator of the amount of iron stored in the body." (Webster's New World Medical Dictionary. 2003).

Hematocrit is defined as "The proportion of the blood that consists of packed red blood cells. The hematocrit is expressed as a percentage by volume. The red cells are packed by centrifugation." (Webster's New World Medical Dictionary. 2003).

Hepcidin is a recently discovered peptide hormone produced by the liver, that appears to be the master regulator of iron homeostasis in humans and other mammals. (Wikipedia 2008)

Transferrin is "A plasma protein that transports iron through the blood to the liver, spleen and bone marrow." (Webster's New World Medical Dictionary. 2003).

Platelet. A platelet is "An irregular, disc-shaped element in the blood that assists in blood clotting. During normal blood clotting, the platelets clump together (aggregate). Although platelets are often classed as blood cells, they are actually fragments of large bone marrow cells called megakaryocytes." (Webster's New World Medical Dictionary. 2003).

Gluten. Gluten is defined as a sub-group of elastic storage proteins in wheat, rye and barley that have been shown to incite immune reactions among those with celiac disease (Braly, Hoggan. 2002).

Storage proteins, as found in wheat, rye, and barley seeds/grains, are defined as groups of proteins that provide nutrients for the germination of that seed/grain (Braly, Hoggan. 2002).

Sickle cell anemia. Sickle cell anemia is "A genetic blood disease due to the presence of an abnormal form of hemoglobin, namely hemoglobin S. Hemoglobin is the molecule in red blood cells that transports oxygen from the lungs to the farthest areas of the body." (Webster's New World Medical Dictionary. 2003).

Thalassemia major. Thalassemia major is "The dire disease also known as beta thalassemia. The clinical picture of this form of anemia was first described in 1925 by the pediatrician Thomas Benton Cooley. Other names for the disease are Cooley's anemia and Mediterranean anemia. The term thalassemia was coined by the Nobel Prize winning pathologist George Whipple and the professor of pediatrics William Bradford at U. of Rochester because thalassa in Greek means the sea (like the Mediterranean Sea) + -emia means in the blood so thalassemia means sea in the blood. Thalassemia is not just one disease. It is a complex contingent of genetic (inherited) disorders all of which involve underproduction of hemoglobin, the indispensable molecule in red blood cells that carries oxygen." (Webster's New World Medical Dictionary. 2003).

Thalassemia minor. Thalassemia minor is "Also called thalassemia trait, thalassemia minor is the carrier state for beta thalassemia. People who are carriers (heterozygotes) have just one thalassemia gene, are said to have thalassemia minor, and are essentially normal." (Webster's New World Medical Dictionary. 2003).

Hemochromatosis. Hemochromatosis is "An inherited disorder in how the body absorbs and stores iron. The excess iron gives the skin a bronze color and damages the liver and other organs. Diabetes is also a part of the syndrome due to damage to the pancreas" (Webster's New World Medical Dictionary. 2003).

Polyphenols are tannic acid which inhibits non-heme iron absorption. (Siegenberg, Baynes, Bothwell, Macfarlane, Lamparelli, Car, MacPhail, Schmidt, Tal, , Mayet, (1991).

Phytate (phytate phosphorous) is an inhibitor of non-heme iron absorption from plants. They are found in abundance in the bran of grains (Cordain, 1999).

Reference range. also called the 'normal range' and it defines the test results that would not usually herald a problem.

It is also important to distinguish between heme iron and non-heme iron.

Heme iron. Heme iron is derived from animal

Non-heme iron, on the other hand, is derived largely from plant foods, and absorption is improved in the presence of vitamin C, malic acid, meat, fish, or poultry. Further, non-heme iron absorption is negatively affected by the presence of other minerals, phytates, oxalate, and tannin, as defined above.

REFERENCES:

1. Ashby, D. (1996). Can iron supplementation improve cognitive functioning? *The Lancet.* 348, 973.

2. Ames, B., (2003). The Metabolic Tune-Up: Metabolic Harmony and Disease Prevention. *The Journal of Nutrition.133, 1544S-1548S.*

3. Beard, J. (2003). Iron Deficiency Alters Brain Development and Functioning. *The Juornal of Nutrition,* 133, 1468S-1472S.

4. Braly, J. and Hoggan, R. (2002). *Dangerous Grains: Why gluten cereal grains may be hazardous to your health, Penguin-Putnam-Avery, N.Y., N.Y..*

5. Bramhagen, A.C., Virtanen, M., Siimes, M.A., Axelsson, I., (2003). Transferrin receptor in children and its correlation with iron status and types of milk consumption. *Acta Paediatr. Jun;92(6):671-5.*

6. Branca, F., and Rossi, L., (2002). The role of fermented milk in complimentary feeding of young children: lessons from transition countries. *European Journal of Clinical Nutrition.* 56, n4S, S16-20.

7. British Columbia Guidelines and Protocols Advisory Committee. (2002). Investigation and Management of Iron Deficiency. *Guidelines & Protocols.* Victoria, B.C., Health Services, British Columbia Provincial Government.

8. Brown, K. (1972). Prevalence of Anemia Among Preadolescent and Young Adolescent Urban Black Americans *Journal of Pediatrics*; 81, 4, 714-718, Oct 72.

9. Bruner, A., Joffe, A., Duggan, A.K., Casella, J.F., Brandt, J., (1996). Randomised study of cognitive effects of iron supplementation in non-anaemic iron-deficient adolescent girls. *Lancet. Oct 12;348(9033):992-6.*

10. Buchannan, G. (1999). The tragedy of iron deficiency during infancy and early childhood. *The Journal of Pediatrics,* 135, 4, 413-415.

11. Butriss, J., (1997). Food and nutrition: attitudes, beliefs, and knowledge in the United Kingdom. *American Journal of Clinical Nutrition. 65, 1985S-1986S.*

12. Caballero, B., (2002). Global patterns of child health: the role of nutrition. *Annals of nutrition & metabolism.. 46 Suppl 1:3-7.*

13. Cavill, I.,(2003). Intravenous iron as adjuvant therapy: a two-edged sword? *Nephrol Dial Transplant. Nov;18 Suppl 8:viii24-8.*

14. Chicago Public Schools (2000). http://intranet.cps.k12.il.us/Assessments/Ideas_and_Rubr ics/Intro_Scoring/intro_scoring.html

15. Cook, D.M. (2002) Iatrogenic illness: a primer for nurses. Dermatol Nurs. Feb;14(1):15-20, 52.

16. Cordain, L., (1999). Cereal grains: humanity's double-edged sword. World Rev Nutr Diet. 84:19-73.

17. Cutler, P., (1991).Iron overload in psychiatric illness. *Am J Psychiatry. Jan;148(1):147-8.*

18. Dagher, A., Owen, A.M., Boecker,H., Brooks, D.J., (2001). The role of the striatum and hippocampus in planning The role of the striatum and hippocampus in A PET activation study in Parkinson's disease. *Brain 124, 1020-1032*

19. Davidsson, L., (2003). Approaches to Improve Iron Bioavailability from Complementary Foods. *The Journal of Nutrition. 133, 1560S.*

20. de Benoist, B., (2001). Iron-Deficiency Anemia: Reexamining the Nature and Magnitude of the Public Health Problem. *Journal of Nutrition. 131, 564S.*

21. Deruisseau, K., Roberts, L., Kushnick, M., Evans, A., Austin, K., Haymes, E.(2004)Iron status of young males

and females performing weight-training exercise Med Sci Sports Exerc. Feb;36(2):241-8.

22. Duhan, A., Khetarpaul N., Bishnoi, S.,(2002). Changes in phytates and HCl extractability of calcium, phosphorus, and iron of soaked, dehulled, cooked, and sprouted pigeon pea cultivar (UPAS-120).Plant Foods Hum Nutr. Fall;57(3-4):275-84.

23. Eisenstein, R., and Ross, K., (2003). Novel Roles for Iron Regulatory Proteins in the Adaptive Response to Iron Deficiency. *The Journal of Nutrition. 133,1510S-1516S.*

24. Fewtrell, L., Pruss-Ustun, A., Landrigan, P., Ayuso-Mateos, J., (2004). Estimating the global burden of disease of mild mental retardation and cardiovascular diseases from environmental lead exposure. *Environ Res. Feb;94(2):120-33.*

25. Fine, K.D., (1996). The prevalence of occult gastrointestinal bleeding in celiac sprue.*N Engl J Med. May 2;334(18):1163-7.*

26. Finefrock, A., Bush, A., Doraiswamy, P., (2003). Current status of metals as therapeutic targets in Alzheimer's disease. *J Am Geriatr Soc. 51(8):1143-8.*

27. Friel, J., Andrews, W., Aziz, K., Kwa, P., Lepage, G., L'Abbe, M., (2001). A randomized trial of two levels of iron supplementation and developmental outcome in low birth weight infants. *Journal of Pediatrics. 139, number2, 254-260.*

28. Gibson RS, Hotz C. 2000. The adequacy of micronutrients in complementary foods. Pediatrics. Nov;106(5):1298-9.

29. Golub, M., Keen, C., Gershwin, M., (2000). Moderate Zinc-Iron Deprivation influences Behavior but not Growth in Adolescent Rhesus Monkeys. *The Journal of Nutrition. 130, 354S-357S.*

30. Gordon, N. (2003) Iron deficiency and the intellect. Brain Dev. 2003 Jan;25(1):3-8.

31. Goswami, T., Rolfs, A., Hediger, M.A., (2002). Iron transport: emerging roles in health and disease. *Biochem Cell Biol. 80(5):679-89.*

32. GrahamR., and Stangoulis, J., (2003). Trace Element Uptake and Distribution in Plants. *The Journal of Nutrition. 133,1502S-1505S.*

33. Grantham-McGregor, S.M., Ani, C.C., (2001). Undernutrition and mental development.

34. Groner JA, Holtzman NA, Charney E, Mellits ED. (1986). A randomized trial of oral iron on tests of short-term memory and attention span in young pregnant women. J Adolesc Health Care. Jan;7(1):44-8.

35. Gropper SS, Blessing D, Dunham K, Barksdale JM.Iron status of female collegiate athletes involved in different sports. Biol Trace Elem Res. 2006 Jan;109(1):1-14.

36. Hadjivassiliou. M., Chattopadhyay, A.K., Davies-Jones, G.A., Gibson, A., Grunewald, R.A., Lobo, A.J., (1997). Neuromuscular disorder as a presenting feature of coeliac disease. J *Neurol Neurosurg Psychiatry. Dec;63(6):770-5.*

37. Hadjivassiliou, M., Davies-Jones, G.A., Sanders, D.S., Grunewald R.A., (2003). Dietary treatment of gluten ataxia. J Neurol Neurosurg Psychiatry. 2003 Sep;74(9):1221-4.

38. Hallberg L, Rossander-Hultén L, Brune M, Gleerup A. (1992)Calcium and iron absorption: mechanism of action and nutritional importance. Eur J Clin Nutr. May; 46(5):317-27.

39. Halterman, J.S., Kaczorowski, J.M., Aligne, C.A., Auinger, P., Szilagyi, P.G., (2001). Iron deficiency and cognitive achievement among school-aged children and adolescents in the United States. Pediatrics. 2001 Jun;107(6):1381-6.

40. Hallberg, L. (1995) Results of surveys to assess iron status in Europe. Nutrition reviews. 11:314-322.

41. Hashizume. M., Shimoda, T., Sasaki, S., Kunii, O., Caypil, W., Dauletbaev, D., Chiba, M., (2004). Anaemia in relation to low bioavailability of dietary iron among school-aged children in the Aral Sea region, Kazakhstan. Int J Food Sci Nutr. Feb;55(1):37-43.

42. Herbert, V., (2001). Letter to the Editor: Hereditary Hemochromatosis. *Ann Intern Med 135 (12): page 1091.*

43. Hercberg, S., Preziosi, P., Galan, P.(2001) Iron deficiency in Europe. Public Health Nutrition 4:537-545.

44. Hiroshi. I., Yoshio, S., Naotaka,H., Akiko, H.,and Mitsumasa O., (2003). The Assay of Ascorbic Acid in Serum Is Not Affected by Physiological Concentrations of Transferrin and Hemoglobin. J*ournal of Nutritional Science and Vitaminology. Vol.49, No.4*

45. Hollan, S., (1996). Iron supplementation and cognitive function. *The Lancet. 348, 1669-1670.*

46. Hoggan, R., (1997). Absolutism's Hidden Message for Medical Scientism. *Interchange. 28, no. 2&3, 183-189*

47. Hua, N.W., Stoohs, R.A., Facchini, F.S., (2001). Low iron status and enhanced insulin sensitivity in lacto-ovo vegetarians. Br J Nutr. 2001 Oct;86(4):515-9.

48. Hurtado, E., Claussen, A., Scott, K., (1999). Early childhood anemia and mild or moderate mental retardation. *American Journal of Clinical Nutrition. 69, 115-119.*

49. Innvista
http://www.innvista.com/health/ailments/anemias/anemc hro.htm

50. Kapil, U., Bhavna, A., (2002). Adverse effects of poor micronutrient status during childhood and adolescence. Nutr Rev. May;60(5 Pt 2):S84-90. Review.

51. Knivsberg, A.M., (1997). Urine patterns, peptide levels and IgA/IgG antibodies to food proteins in children with dyslexia. *Pediatr Rehabil. Jan-Mar;1(1):25-33.*

52. Krebs, N., (2000). Dietary Zinc and Iron Sources, Physical Growth and Cognitive Development of Breastfed Infants. *The Journal of Nutrition. 130, 358S-360S.*

53. Krechnmer, N., Beard, J., Carlson, S., (1996). The role of nutrition in the development of normal cognition. *American Journal of Clinical Nutrition. 63, 997S-1001S.*

54. Layrisse, M., Garcia-Casal, M., Solano, L., Baron, M., Arguello, F., Llovera, D., Ramirez, J., Leets, I., Tropper, E., (2000). Iron bioavailability in humans from breakfasts enriched with iron bis-glycine chelate, phytates and polyphenols. J Nutr. Sep;130(9):2195-9. Erratum in: J Nutr 2000 Dec;130(12):3106.

55. Leibel, R.L. (1977). Behavioral and biochemical correlates of iron deficiency. Journal of the American Dietetic Association.. Oct;71(4):398-404.

56. Liu, J., Raine, A., Venables, P., Dalais, C., Mednick, S., (2003). Malnutrition at Age 3 Years and Lower Cognitive Ability at Age 11 Years. *Archives of Pediatrics & Adolescent Medicine. 157, 93600.*

57. Liu, Y., Reichelt, K., (2001). A serotonin uptake-stimulating tetra-peptide found in urines from ADHD children. *World J Biol Psychiatry. Jul;2(3):144-8.*

58. Logan, S., Martins, S., Gilbert, R., (2001). Iron therapy for improving psychomotor development and cognitive function in children under the age of three with iron deficiency anaemia. *Cochrane Database Syst Rev. (2):CD001444.*

59. Lombardo, F., Salzano, G., Messina, M.F., De Luca, F.. (2003) How self management therapy can improve

quality of life for diabetic patients. *Acta Biomed Ateneo Parmense. 74 Suppl 1:26-8.*

60. Lozoff, B., Jimenez, E., Hagen, J., Mollen, E.., Wolf, A., (2000). Poorer Behavioral and Developmental Outcome More than 10 Years After Treatment for Iron Deficiency in Infancy. *Pediatrics. 105, number 4, 1-11.*

61. Lynch, S., (1997). Interaction of Iron with Other Nutrients. *Nutrition Reviews, 55, 4, 102-109.*

62. Marinaro, M., Fasano, A., DeMagistris, M., (2003). Zonula Occludens Toxin Acts as an Adjuvant through Different Mucosal Routes and Induces Protective Immune Responses. *Infection and Immunity. 71, 4, 1897-1902.*

63. McCullough, M., Feskanich, D., Rimm, E.B., Giovannucci, E.L., Ascherio, A., Variyam, J.N., Spiegelman, D., Stampfer, M.J., Willett, W.C.. (2000). Adherence to the Dietary Guidelines for Americans and risk of major chronic disease in men. Am J Clin Nutr. 2000 Nov;72(5):1223-31.

64. Mofidi, S., (2003). Nutritional Management of Pediatric Food Hypersensitivity. *Pediatrics 11, number 6, 1645-1653.*

65. Naveh, Y., Shalata, A., Shenker, L., Coleman, R., (2000). Absorption of iron in rats with experimental enteritis. *Biometals. Mar;13(1):29-35.*

66. Nelson, C., Erikzon, K., Pinero, D., Beard, J., (1997). In Vivo Dopamine Metabolism is Altered in Iron-Deficient Anemic Rats. *Journal of Nutrition. 127, 282-2288.*

67. Nestle, M., (1993). Dietary Advice for the 1990s: The Political History of the Food Guide Pyramid. Caduceus Winter IX: 3.

68. Nestle Nutr Workshop Ser Clin Perform Programme. (5):1-14; discussion 14-8.

69. Otero, G.A., Aguirre, D.M., Porcayo, R., Fernandez, T. (1999). Psychological and electroencephalographic study in school children with iron deficiency. The International journal of neuroscience.. Aug;99(1-4):113-21.

70. Palti, H., Meijer, A., Adler, B. (1985). Learning achievement and behavior at school of anemic and non-anemic infants. Early human development.. Jan;10(3-4):217-223.

71. Penland, J., (2000). Behavioral Data and Methodology Issues in Studies of Zinc Nutrition in Humans. *Journal of Nutrition. 130, 361s-364s.*

72. Pettifor, J., (2001). Iron deficiency and impaired child development. BMJ. December 323; 1378-1379.

73. Pilu, R., Panzeri, D., Gavazzi, G., Rasmussen, S., Consonni, G., Nielsen, E.,(2003). Phenotypic, genetic and molecular characterization of a maize low phytic acid mutant (lpa241).Theor Appl Genet. 2003 Oct;107(6):980-7. Epub Oct 02.

74. Pollitt, E. (1994). Poverty and Child Development: Relevance of Research in Developing Countries to the United States. *Child Development*; v65 n2 Apr p283-95

75. Pollitt, E., (1997). Iron Deficiency and Educational Deficiency. *Nutrition Reviews, 55, no. 4, 133-140.*

76. Pollitt, E., (2001). The Developmental and Probablistic Nature of the Functional Consequences of Iron-Deficiency Anemia in Children. *Journal of Nutrition. 131, 669s-675s.*

77. Ragozzino, M.E., Choi, D. (2004). Dynamic changes in acetylcholine output in the medial striatum during place reversal learning. Learn Mem. 2004 Jan-Feb;11(1):70-7.

78. Rajakumar, K., (2000). Pellagra in the United States: a historical perspective. *South Med J. Mar;93(3):272-7.*

79. Rettmer, R., Carlson, T., Origenes, M., Jack, R., Labbe, R., (1999). Zinc Protoporphyrin/Heme Ratio for

Diagnosis of Preanemic Iron Deficiency. *Pediatrics. 104, no.3, 104.*

80. Roe, D. (1973). *A Plague of Corn. Ithaca and London. Cornell University Press.*

81. Roebothan BV, Chandra RK.The contribution of dietary iron to iron status in a group of elderly subjects. Int J Vitam Nutr Res. 1996;66(1):66-70.

82. Rogers JL, Kesner RP. Cholinergic modulation of the hippocampus during encoding and retrieval of tone/shock-induced fear conditioning. Learn Mem. 2004 Jan-Feb;11(1):102-7.

83. Rogers, I., Emmett, P., (2001). Fat Content of the Diet A,pg Preschool Children in Southwest Britain: II. Relationship With Growth, Blood Lipids, and Iron Status. Pediatrics. 108, no. 3, 108.

84. Sandstead, H., (2000). Causes of Iron and Zinc Deficiencies and Their Effects on Brain. *Journal of Nutrition. 130, 347s-349s.*

85. Saloojee, H., Pettifor, J., (2001). Iron deficiency and impaired child development. *British Medical Journal. 323, 377-1378.*

86. Samuelson G, Bratteby LE, Enghardt H, Hedgren M. 2000. Food habits and energy and nutrient intake in Swedish adolescents approaching the year *Acta Paediatr Suppl. 1996 Sep;415:1-19.*

87. Santucci, A.C., Cardiello, J. (2004). Memory Reactivation in Rats Treated With the 5-HT-sub-1-sub(A) Agonist 8-OHDP AT: A Case of Gone, but Not Forgotten. *Behav Neurosci. Feb;118(1):248-52.*

88. Siegenberg, D., Baynes, R.D., Bothwell, T.H., Macfarlane, B.J., Lamparelli, R.D., Car, N.G., MacPhail, P., Schmidt, U., Tal, A., Mayet, F., (1991). Ascorbic acid prevents the dose-dependent inhibitory effects of polyphenols and phytates on nonheme-iron absorption. *Am J Clin Nutr. 1991 Feb;53(2):537-41.*

89. Sobotka, T.J., Whittaker, P., Sobotka, J.M., Brodie, R.E., Quander, D.Y., Robl, M., Bryant, M., Barton, C.N. (1996). Neurobehavioral dysfunctions associated with dietary iron overload. Physiology & behavior.. Feb;59(2):213-9.

90. Solomons, N., (1997). Daily Versus Weekly Iron: We Still Might Not Be Asking the Right Questions. *Nutrition Reviews. 55, no. 4, 141-142.*

91. Stevens, R.D., (2000). Anaemia -- the scourge of the Third World. *Health Millions. Mar-Apr;26(2):21-3.*

92. Stoltzfus, R., (2001). Defining Iron-Deficiency Anemia in Public Health Terms: A Time for Reflection. *Journal of Nutrition. 131, 565s-567s.*

93. Stoltzfus, R.J., Kvalsvig, J.D., Chwaya, HM., Montresor, A., Albonico, M., Tielsch, J.M, Savioli, L., Pollitt, E., (2001). Effects of iron supplementation and anthelmintic treatment on motor and language development of preschool children in Zanzibar: double blind, placebo controlled study. *BMJ. 2001 Dec 15;323(7326):1389-93.*

94. Suh, S.W., Aoyama, K., Chen, Y., Garnier, P., Matsumori, Y., Gum, E., Liu, J., Swanson, R.A. (2003). Hypoglycemic neuronal death and cognitive impairment are prevented by poly(ADP-ribose) polymerase inhibitors administered after hypoglycemia. J Neurosci. Nov 19;23(33):10681-90.

95. Swanson, C.A., (2003). Iron intake and regulation: implications for iron deficiency and iron overload. *Alcohol. Jun;30(2):99-102.*

96. Swartz-Basile, D.A., Goldblatt, M.I., Blaser, C., Decker, P.A., Ahrendt, S.A., Sarna, S.K., Pitt, H.A., (2000). Iron deficiency diminishes gallbladder neuronal nitric oxide synthase. J Surg Res. May 1;90(1):26-31.

97. Thane, C.W., Bates, C.J., Prentice, A.. (2003). Risk factors for low iron intake and poor iron status in a

national sample of British young people aged 4-18 years. *Public Health Nutr. Aug;6(5):485-96.*

98. Theil, E., (2003). Ferritin: At the Crossroads of Iron and Oxygen Metabolism. *Journal of Nutrition. 133, 1549s-1553s.*

99. Thompson, K., Shoham, S., Connor, J., (2001). Iron and neurodegenerative disorders. *Brain Research Bulletin.* 55, Issue 2, 155-164.

100.   Timmann, D, Dimitrova, A, Hein-Kropp, C, Wilhelm, H, Dorfler, A. (2003). Cerebellar agenesis: clinical, neuropsychological and MR findings. Neurocase. 2003 Oct;9(5):402-13.

101.   Tseng, M., Chakraborty, H., Robinson, D., Mendez, M., Kohlmeier, L.,(1997). Adjustment of iron intake for dietary enhancers and inhibitors in population studies: bioavailable iron in rural and urban residing Russian women and children. J Nutr. Aug;127(8):1456-68.

102.   Walker, A., Walker, B., (1996). Iron supplementation and cognitive function. *The Lancet. 348, 1669.*

103.   Walker, A., (1996). Iron deficiency, development, and cognitive function. *American Journal of Clinical Nutritio. 64, 120-121*

104.   Webb, T.E. & Oski, F.A.(1973). Iron deficiency anemia and scholastic achievement in young adolescents. *Journal of Pediatrics,* 82(5), 827-30.

105.   Webster's New World Medical Dictionary. (2003). Wiley Publishing, Inc. accessed via http://www.medicinenet.com

106.   Willett, W. (2002). *Eat, Drink, and Be Healthy: The Harvard Medical School Guide to Healthy Eating.* Simon & Schuster, N.Y., N.Y.

107.   Willows ND, Dewailly E, Gray-Donald K. (2000) Anemia and iron status in Inuit infants from northern Quebec. Can J Public Health. Nov-Dec;91(6):407-10.

108.   Wolf, F.M., Guevara, J.P., Grum, C.M., Clark, N.M., Cates, C.J. (2003). Educational interventions for asthma in children. *Cochrane Database Syst Rev. 2003;(1):CD000326.*

109.   Wolfe, Patricia. (2001) Brain Matters. ASCD, Alexandria, VA.

110.   Yehuda, S., & Rabinovitz, S.,(2001) Importance of brain iron to the pregnant mother and the infant.: Nutrition in the female life cycle. ISAS INternational Seminars Ltd. P.O. Box 34001, Jerusalem 91340, Israel

111.   Yu, S., Kogan, M., Gergen, P., (1997). Vitamin-Mineral Supplement Use Among Preschool Children in the United States. Pediatrics 100, no. 5, 100.

112.   Zimmermann M.B., Hess, S.Y., Molinari, L., De Benoist, B., Delange, F., Braverman, L.E., Fujieda, K, Ito, Y., Jooste, P.L., Moosa, K., Pearce, E.N., Pretell, E.A., Shishiba, Y. (2004). New reference values for thyroid volume by ultrasound in iodine-sufficient schoolchildren: a World Health Organization/Nutrition for Health and Development Iodine Deficiency Study Group Report. Am J Clin Nutr. Feb;79(2):231-7.

113.   Zlotkin, S., (2003). Clinical nutrition: 8. The role of nutrition in the prevention of iron deficiency anemia in infants, children, and adolescents. *Canadian Medical Association Journal. 168, no. 1, 59-63.*

Appendix A:

Iron Information Resources

Internet – Medscape, PubMed

Library – popular books, medical newsletters, peer-reviewed journals, health magazines, etc.

The Merck Manual

WHO publications for medical/epidemiological data and information

Codex Alimentarius publications for nutritional issues

USDA – although some researchers have pointed out the conflict of interests inherent in the USDA's dual mandate of promoting agricultural interests while providing nutritional advice to the customers of this industry.